THE

MIND-BODY

FERTILITY

CONNECTION

ABOUT THE AUTHOR

James Schwartz, BCH, is a board-certified hypnotherapist and an NLP practitioner. He is certified by the National Guild of Hypnotists and a member of the Colorado Association of Psychotherapists. James is the founder and director of the Rocky Mountain Hypnotherapy Center in Lakewood, Colorado, and is certified in Complementary Medical Hypnosis, NeuroLinguistic Programming, and HypnoBirthing®. Through his extensive hypnotherapy work with infertility clients, James created and developed a highly successful fertility program called *Hypnosis to Promote Fertility* which focuses on healing the mental and emotional barriers that can often prevent conception. This work became the basis for *The Mind-Body Fertility Connection.*

James has published several articles about using the mind-body connection to promote fertility; facilitated educational seminars for women who struggle with infertility; and was invited to present an overview of his *Hypnosis to Promote Fertility* program to the National Guild of Hypnotists at their 2006 convention. More information about this program can be found at *www.rmhypnotherapy.com.*

James is a graduate of California State University at Dominguez Hills and San Diego State University. He is a former teacher of English, ESL (USA and Japan), and writing for multimedia, and he has taught courses in stress management and meditation.

JAMES SCHWARTZ

THE

MIND - BODY

FERTILITY

CONNECTION

THE TRUE PATHWAY TO CONCEPTION

Llewellyn Publications
Woodbury, Minnesota

First Edition
First Printing, 2008

Cover art leaf image © by DataCraft/Imagenavi/Punchstock
Cover design by Kevin R. Brown
Interior illustrations by Mary Ann Zapalac
Llewellyn is a registered trademark of Llewellyn Worldwide, Ltd.

Library of Congress Cataloging-in-Publication Data

Schwartz, Jim (James), 1957-
  The mind-body fertility connection : the true pathway to conception /
Jim Schwartz. —1st ed.
      p. cm.
  Includes bibliographical references and index.
  ISBN 978-0-7387-1376-2
  1. Infertility, Female—Psychological aspects—Popular works. 2. Conception—
Psychological aspects—Popular works. 3. Infertility, Female—Alternative treatment—
Popular works. 4. Mind and body therapies—Popular works. I. Title.
RG201.S39   2008
618.1'78—dc22   2008007961

Llewellyn Publications
A Division of Llewellyn Worldwide, Ltd.
2143 Wooddale Drive, Dept. 978-0-7387-1376-2
Woodbury, Minnesota 55125-2989, U.S.A.
www.llewellyn.com

Printed in the United States of America

CONTENTS

ACKNOWLEDGMENTS

The most important person I want to acknowledge in helping me prepare this book is also the most important person in my life, my wife, Julie. Not only has she given much input into the writing and editing of this book, but she has also been a loving and supportive companion. I am grateful to have her inspiration and light in my life. As a practitioner of Eastern medicine who specializes in fertility work, Julie served as a consultant for the acupuncture information in this book.

I want to express appreciation to the many practitioners, especially the acupuncturists—including Linda Marler—with whom I have worked. I believe it is our combined effort that has created such incredible success with fertility and in many other areas of holistic healing.

To the women who graciously agreed to share their personal stories in this book, I would like to extend my gratitude. Those stories have enriched this material while providing guidance and encouragement for women who are searching for different approaches to embracing their own fertility.

I want to thank Dr. Elizabeth Muir for our ongoing correspondence and her support in this field. Through her efforts, and the efforts of Philip Quinn, the application of hypnosis for fertility has become a reality.

Two of my writing teachers deserve special mention for their encouragement and support: Minas Savvas and Hal Marienthal.

Jerry Kein, who has been a leader in the field of hypnosis, should be recognized for his efforts to enlighten, inspire, and encourage hypnotists around the world.

Finally, I would like to thank the people at Llewellyn Worldwide, including Carrie Obry, for their interest and support of the book and in this subject which is so important to millions of people who are searching for answers to help them on this journey.

INTRODUCTION

Millions of women around the world—including over seven million in the United States alone—have been diagnosed with "unexplained infertility." This condition has driven the pharmaceutical and medical industries to focus on biologically manipulating the body to create life.

The Mind-Body Fertility Connection asks a different question about the reasons for infertility: if there is no physiological explanation for the condition, then could the answers exist in the mental and emotional realms, buried in the subconscious minds of women who struggle to conceive? After all, scientific studies have now proven that a woman has a better chance of conceiving if she uses a mind-body program than if she undergoes a $20,000 in vitro procedure.

This book unveils a new pathway to conception: a pathway of healing through the emotions which allows women to unblock the potential for childbearing. This book dissects the feelings, beliefs, and old emotional injuries that often create subconscious obstacles that can disrupt an otherwise healthy functioning reproductive system. Taking a closer look at this connection from a mental/emotional standpoint broadens our treatment options and our ability to achieve greater success.

In my practice, I work with infertility clients every day. Years ago, I created and developed one of the first programs in the United States that was specifically designed to work with the mental and emotional components of infertility. As I did more and more of this work, it became apparent that many common emotional factors were expressed by fertility clients, and only after addressing these issues did they conceive. This, I believe, is an important, unexplored piece of the infertility puzzle, one that holds the true secrets for successful conception. As a board-certified hypnotherapist and the creator of the *Hypnosis to Promote Fertility* program, I specialize in working with the subconscious mind, which is where much of the essential information regarding infertility is stored. Few people work as intimately with the subconscious mind as a hypnotherapist, and this process, I believe, holds the potential to explain what has often been labeled as unexplained.

Some people in the traditional medical and psychiatric communities may not agree with my perspectives and opinions, but with infertility at epidemic proportions, the conventional methods and treatments practiced over the last ten to fifteen years have proven to be costly and largely inefficient. If that disagreement creates dialogue, then this book has been successful, because new approaches are long overdue.

Within this book, I provide interactive opportunities for readers to help identify and work through some of the potential blocks that might be interfering with conception. I also provide an action plan to help guide women through the process of getting their minds and bodies ready to conceive, including information about alternative therapies and traditional treatments set within a timeline so that readers can plan what steps to take in order to maximize their chances of becoming pregnant. They say that knowledge is power, and my goal in writing *The Mind-Body Fertility Connection* is to encourage women to explore the wisdom buried within themselves and experience their fertility as a journey of empowerment.

CHAPTER ONE

THE FERTILITY JOURNEY

You've been there before—perhaps dozens of times. The ovulation indicator shows you are nearing your surge, and what started out to be a sense of excitement in your body has come to be replaced by an unmistakable feeling of tension and foreboding. A million thoughts and feelings swirl through your mind and body: "Will I be able to conceive this time?" "Why is this so difficult?" "Am I unworthy to bear a child?" "Why is it that everyone else can get pregnant but me?" "Did I wait too long?" "Am I too old?" "Why is it that I can be successful at everything else I do, but not this?" "What is everyone going to think if I can't get pregnant?"

These are some of the heartfelt emotions expressed by my fertility clients, women who are frustrated and grief-stricken by the inability to conceive, women who are asking the question: could there be something else in my psyche that might have been overlooked in the standard approaches to treating infertility?

Millions of women are struggling with the dilemma of diagnoses that have been handed them: "unexplained infertility" or "old eggs" or "high FSH (follicle-stimulating hormone score)." The one-size-fits-all solutions that are proposed include stimulation drugs, intrauterine insemination (a technique, commonly referred to as an IUI, where sperm is injected through a flexible catheter directly into the uterus), in vitro fertilization (a medical technique, commonly referred to as an IVF, where follicles are retrieved from a woman's body, fertilized with sperm in a laboratory, and then the fertilized eggs are put back into a woman's uterus), donor eggs, and medical treatments and procedures that feel unnatural. These come with a very high price tag and often fail. For the woman who feels that this is simply not what she can embrace either morally, physically, financially, or emotionally, too few alternatives have been available.

My first infertility client told me the same story that I've heard hundreds of times since that day: she had been told by a fertility specialist that she would never conceive naturally due to poor egg quality, but she could undergo an IVF procedure with fertility drugs, artificial hormones, and donor eggs, and then she would have a fairly good chance of having a baby. This particular client didn't want to use drugs or medical procedures or donor eggs. She wanted to conceive naturally and have a baby her own way.

So, we started her program by reducing stress through meditation. We worked with a visualizing process where she created the conception in her mind. We incorporated mind-body healing techniques that were based on both Eastern and Western medicine, and most importantly, we focused on identifying and processing the deep-seated issues that appeared to be interfering with conception for her.

After a few sessions her outlook changed: she believed in herself and that she could have a baby. Three months after she started working with me, she was pregnant naturally. Nine months after that, she had an amazing baby boy.

Since then, there has been a steady stream of people coming to work on their infertility, and as I worked with them, I began to notice patterns and trends. First and foremost, women struggling with infertility needed someone who believed in them and could be there for support. Many of the women had lost much of their confidence and self-esteem. Many of them felt defeated and no longer believed they could get pregnant. Many of them felt that they were letting everyone—husbands, families, in-laws—down. Many of them had been discouraged and incredibly saddened by the diagnoses they had received from their doctors. Many of them felt like for the first time in their lives they had failed at something they never imagined would be difficult. Many of them were blaming themselves and their infertility on things that they had done or experienced in their past. Many of them were putting intense pressure on themselves to try to somehow make this happen. Many of them talked about the sadness or depression that was becoming more and more difficult to overcome. Many of them were on the verge of giving up hope. Many of them were in a state of extreme stress because of the invasive tests, techniques, procedures, and constant appointments. Many were simply heartbroken.

What I saw was a million emotions that had been building up during their struggle, with no one there to help them heal those emotional wounds. Since the popular belief has always been that emotions have nothing to do with one's ability to conceive, what these women were given was more tests, more procedures, more drugs, more expenses, and more feelings of frustration and defeat. In essence, they were being told that their feelings and emotions were not important—but something about that message didn't feel right.

In the past, the medical community has acknowledged that stress and anxiety can be at the root of myriad physical disharmonies including migraine headaches, heart disease, high blood pressure, irritable bowel issues, acid reflux, skin rashes, and insomnia. When it came to infertility, however, the medical community generally took the position that the ability to conceive and carry full-term was strictly a physiological process and the mind and emotions had nothing to do with it.

Infertility is *not* simply a physical issue, and it's time to acknowledge the need to address the mental and emotional components that play a vital role in creating conception. Feelings, emotions, fears, frustrations, anxieties, and stressors are all major factors in this very complicated process.

When the emotional issues connected to infertility are examined, the mind-body relationship becomes very apparent. Take the woman who has had a couple of miscarriages and is consumed with the fear of losing another baby. Should she believe that her feelings aren't important and her emotional state has nothing to do with her infertility? What about the woman who experienced sexual abuse early in her life and is now unable to let her body relax, let alone be in a place of trust? Don't her feelings count, and could those feelings be related to her inability to conceive? What about the woman who was told by her doctor that she has a very slim chance of ever conceiving naturally? Does that information have any effect on her outlook and does her negative outlook have anything to do with success or failure? Should the woman diagnosed with unexplained infertility—meaning that there is no physiological cause—be told that whatever feelings and emotional issues she has are not relevant? How does it feel when one is told that their emotions aren't important because the conception process is nothing more than a matter of biological functions? All of these feelings, emotions, and issues *are* part of the infertility picture and they *do* need to be acknowledged and addressed. Dr. Alice Domar, an assistant professor at Harvard Medical School and a leader in the field of infertility research, observed this about women struggling to conceive: "infertile women report equivalent levels of anxiety and depression as [do] women with cancer, HIV status, or heart disease."[1]

The connection between emotional issues and infertility is not a completely new concept. Chapter 2 of this book contains several studies, conducted over the last two decades, providing scientific evidence that there is a powerful connection between mind-body work and one's ability to conceive. Unfortunately, many people have been unaware of the research supporting this connection. Others may have suspected that the emotional state might be related to the inability to conceive, but they didn't know what to do about it. Unfortunately, there are some, with an awareness of this connection, who have chosen to look the other way.

This book is about educating and presenting a different perspective. Readers who want a scientific overview that discusses physiology and medically assisted reproductive techniques (ART) should seek out a book on that subject written by a doctor. People who want the traditional psychotherapeutic overview about infertility can find books written from that perspective. The audience for this book is the person who wants to follow a different path. Scientific studies (presented in chapter two of this book) are now showing that when it comes to fertility, the alternative modalities that promote the mind-body connection have been producing better results than traditional allopathic medicine. Dr.

Randine Lewis, who specializes in acupuncture to treat infertility, had this to say about Western medical treatments for infertility:

> Unfortunately, [while] we hear a great deal about how Western reproductive medicine has helped women conceive, we hear a great deal *less* about the pain, expense, and statistically low success rates of such procedures. Research shows that even young women using IVF techniques have between a 20 and 30 percent chance of conceiving. The chances fall to less than 10 percent for women at age thirty-nine and only 3 percent for women at age forty-four. On average, women go through seven cycles of ART before they either conceive or quit, spending tens to hundreds of thousands of dollars in their attempts to have children.[2]

That isn't to say that allopathic medicine can't be beneficial with infertility. It can be, especially in situations such as helping to identify hidden physical problems. But the very diagnosis of "unexplained infertility," given to seven million women in the United States alone, is the medical community's way of saying that there is nothing *physically* wrong that is getting in the way of conception. If the physiology is not the problem, then we need to look at the mental and emotional realms to determine whether the cause of the infertility might lie there. Two decades of research (see chapter two) have made a statement about infertility: the mind-body connection *is* a vital component in the conception process and it is time to acknowledge and address that work as an integral part of treating infertility.

Addressing the mind-body connection involves working with the subconscious mind. That is where all of our issues, our feelings, our emotions, our fears and anxieties, our life experiences, our behavioral patterns, and our beliefs are stored. Negative feelings and emotions within the subconscious can intensify and become all-consuming to the woman experiencing infertility. In order to make lasting changes in our lives, the changes—or healing—need to occur at the subconscious level. That subconscious healing has the potential to unlock one's ability to conceive. (The inner workings of the subconscious mind and an overview of how the mind works are discussed in chapter 3.)

This book addresses the mind-body connection to fertility. It may be the most important—and most overlooked—factor in achieving conception. This book dissects the feelings, emotions, beliefs, and blocks that need to be healed in order for one to become pregnant, and it looks at how those obstacles can be overcome. It is information that every woman on this journey needs to know.

After years of doing hypnotherapy work to promote conception, I have gained much insight into the subconscious programming of women who have been struggling to conceive. I learned about the feelings and emotions in the minds of infertility clients, and I learned what they needed to process and heal. The diagnosis of "unexplained infertility" created a genuine need for women to have an outlet for emotional healing, a different kind of healing that has not been available within the framework of the standard approaches to working with infertility.

People always want to know what kind of success I've had in this area. In the past, I have always referred them to the scientific studies (included in chapter two of this book). Those are the official numbers that one should reference when evaluating this work. My numbers are not scientific. There was no double blind or control group with my clients. I simply kept records, over the course of several years, of each of the clients I have worked with, whether or not they became pregnant, and whether or not they carried full term. The average age of the women that I saw during that timeframe was 36.9. Of the clients I saw who had been tested for a follicle-stimulating hormone (FSH), 74 percent had FSH levels that were above 10. A follicle-stimulating hormone or FSH level of ten or above is generally considered by Western medical doctors to be the point where assisted reproductive technology [ART] is necessary, and it is unlikely a woman can conceive naturally once her FSH reaches that threshold. (See chapter 4 for a more detailed discussion of FSH.) The results, while using my *Hypnosis to Promote Fertility* program, were a 60 percent take-home baby rate. Those numbers were not my success rates: they were a reflection of the successes of the women who had done the work. They deserve the credit and the success belongs to them.

It is also important to attribute much of the success in this area to the network of gifted healers who were a part of this process. Most of the clients that I saw during that timeframe worked with an acupuncturist, and many had chosen to add Maya abdominal massage—a gentle, external massage process designed to make sure that the uterus is in proper alignment—as an alternative modality. (See chapter thirteen for more information about alternative modalities.) Each healer in the journey brought their own gifts and talents to the process, and the cumulative efforts of everyone involved created an exponential effect.

Some of the successful clients used Western medical techniques such as intrauterine insemination (IUI) or in vitro procedures (IVF), while others chose to become pregnant by using natural or holistic techniques.

It is important to note that I saw everyone who expressed the desire to do this work. I believe that everyone has the right to explore all options that might help them succeed. My focus was not on the numbers: it was on helping the individual. I have seen women in their late forties, women with follicle-stimulating hormone (FSH) scores in the eighties, women with premature ovarian failure (POF) and polycystic ovarian syndrome (PCOS) who hadn't had periods for over a year. This is a journey about healing and everyone is entitled to have that opportunity, without judgment of their age, history, or diagnostic labels that might have been placed upon them.

This book begins with a look at the studies that support mind-body work and its relationship to conception. Chapter three includes a closer look at the inner workings of the subconscious and an explanation of how the mind works. In many of the subsequent chapters, I talk about emotional blocks and provide exercises and meditations that may offer some relief and insight. That is simply a starting point. There is no replacement for working with someone who can help process and heal the underlying issues.

It is important that everyone reading this book understand that I am not a medical doctor, nor am I a doctor of psychology. I have tried to be as accurate as possible in my descriptions, but be sure to consult with your doctor or an expert in the field to get the definitive answers to your specific health questions. None of the material presented here is intended to be a substitute for traditional medicine. Instead, this work should be viewed as a complementary modality.

In my view, the magical key to unlocking fertility is healing and processing the information deep in the subconscious mind. Whether your goal is to try to conceive naturally or work with assisted reproductive techniques, addressing the subconscious material is probably the most important part of achieving conception. This book is about harnessing the power of the subconscious and utilizing the mind-body connection in a positive way in order to achieve fertility.

STORIES TOLD IN THEIR OWN WORDS

Throughout this book, I include stories from women who went through this process and graciously agreed to share their experiences in order to help others. The act of collecting these stories was simply allowing the women to express their own experiences *in their own words*. All of the stories are from clients with whom I worked, and who had used mind-body modalities on their fertility journeys. Naturally, fictitious names were used to protect identities. The ages of the women who tell their stories ranged from thirty-six to forty-five at the time they began working with hypnosis, with the exception of one woman who was in her late twenties.

In selecting the stories to include in the book, I tried to present a cross-section of women who pursued different strategies to address their situations. Some chose only holistic modalities to support a natural pregnancy while others chose to work with Western medical procedures. Mind-body work is beneficial regardless of whether a woman wants to create a natural pregnancy or use assisted reproductive technology.

The first of these stories, written by Michelle, is important because it shows how alternative modalities can open new doors and offer additional support. Michelle embraced the power of the mind-body connection and discovered that working with the subconscious mind not only made a profound change in her thought processes, but it helped her create the outcome that she had desired.

Michelle's Story
Alternatives to the Western Route

I had been trying to get pregnant for over a year when I went to a reproductive endocrinologist who did a series of tests and found that there was nothing wrong with me, except that my FSH was "ominously" high, at 17. He recommended donor eggs, due to my "mature maternal age" of forty-five. He asked if I had a younger sister or friend who might be willing to donate an egg and also referred me to an agency for egg donation.

I decided I didn't want to go through the typical Western medical route of having an in vitro procedure. My husband suggested I see his friend who was a traditional Chinese practitioner specializing in endocrinology. The first thing the practitioner did was check my adrenal glands with a saliva test which showed that my adrenals were not producing enough precursors for making a sufficient amount of estrogen. Basically, it was Mother Nature's way of saying "this woman is so stressed out she can't possibly deal with another pregnancy." So he gave me some adrenal supplements and told me to change my lifestyle. I cut out all of the caffeine, started doing yoga, and concentrated on decreasing the stress in my life, both mentally and physically.

He then referred me to another traditional Chinese medicine practitioner who gave me herbal teas to take twice a day. I got acupuncture treatments from her once a week. She asked many questions that seemed unusual, but in the Chinese medicine system, it gave her an idea of where I was depleted or weak. She also referred me for Maya uterine massage, which I did once a month.

During the uterine massage, they discovered that my uterus was tilted to the right side. It was interesting because a month earlier, when I had gone in for my hysterosalpingogram (HSG)—

where they check the fallopian tubes for blockages—the radiologist could not get the dye into the right side. She kept telling me to turn over on the table because she was having trouble accessing the right fallopian tube. I was amazed that a month later this young woman who was massaging my uterus was telling me that the uterus tilting off to the right side might be pinching off the fallopian tube. I realized that this is why they couldn't get the dye into my right side.

I was referred to hypnotherapy by the woman who performed the uterine massage. The hypnotherapy part was especially powerful. In my sessions I was told I had to do a meditation every day: it was not enough to just come to weekly sessions, I was supposed to work on this every day. So, every day at work, I would go into my office and shut the door and do the meditation for ten minutes, envisioning the entire conception, and ending each meditation with "I am pregnant, and I am so happy to have this baby."

When the hypnotherapist suggested that at first, I looked at him and said, "I *am* pregnant?" and he said to never use future tense. At the time, I was skeptical, but after doing it, I realized it was a very powerful affirmation. I believe that really helped a lot. I will never forget the time when my subconscious mind really kicked in with that belief. I was driving and heard an advertisement on the radio that said the Rolling Stones were coming to town in several months. My first thought was, "I've got to get tickets," but my next thought was, "I can't go, I'll be pregnant then." Then, my third thought was, "Wow, where did that come from?" It came right out of my subconscious. "No, I'm not going to go: I'm going to be pregnant then." I was convinced. It came out so spontaneously, and that's when I realized how all the meditation and positive affirmations really worked.

All of this work I was doing happened in just four months. It snowballed: one thing led to another to another and another. All these doors kept opening. Outside of traditional Chinese medicine, I didn't know that these other alternatives were available. I found this fascinating because, being in medicine myself, a regis-tered nurse, and having a husband who is a physician, we ended up going with this whole alternative route. I found it ironic that, with both of us working in Western medicine, we shunned that and went a different way.

After four months of this, I became pregnant. I was so shocked, because it had happened so quickly, that I took four pregnancy tests. I now have a beautiful daughter who is seven-teen months old.

I'm sure my pregnancy was a combination of everything I did, but the mind-body work was really amazing. I've told this story several times to my colleagues, and I think this helped them too, knowing I was able to become pregnant naturally at forty-five.

WORKS CITED

1. Alice D. Domar. *The Journal of Psychosomatic Obstetrics and Gynecology* 14, Suppl. (1993): 45–52.
2. Randine Lewis. *The Infertility Cure* (New York: Little, Brown and Company, 2004), 5.

CHAPTER TWO

THE EVIDENCE SUPPORTING THE MIND–BODY CONNECTION

Many clients that I see present some minor physical issues: a small amount of scarring from endometriosis, a fibroid that was removed two years ago, an FSH of 12 (to see why this may not necessarily be a major physical block, see the information in chapter 4 about the stress response), but in most cases, those issues are not enough to prevent conception. The most common profile in infertility—based on observations I've made in my practice—is a woman who presents one or two minor physical concerns, but essentially falls into the "unexplained infertility" diagnosis.

The "unexplained infertility" term raises questions about how much power and influence the mind and the emotions have in the conception process. Can the mind-body connection really affect fertility? Several scientific studies have addressed that question, and the majority of those studies support the belief that the mind-body connection is a vital part of the conception process.

The first study on this topic—which wasn't specifically an infertility study, but rather a look at psychosomatic behavior in general—took place back in the 1970s. Doctors Howard and Martha Lewis, in a book called *Psychosomatics*, studied and documented case studies in which mental and emotional issues affected the condition of the physical body.[1]

One of the case studies described in *Psychosomatics* was an infertility patient whom they referred to as Rena. She was twenty-three years old and really wanted to start a family. The doctors noted that Rena was always saying, "There's nothing I want so much as a baby."[2] Even though Rena wanted a child, she had a great deal of fear around pregnancy. She had heard stories about the dangers and complications of pregnancy, and the anxiety that this created was affecting her to the extent that the doctors observed that Rena's "involuntary nervous system expressed her buried fear by keeping her from becoming pregnant."[3] In other words, Rena's body was having a physical reaction to her fear, and that physical reaction was blocking her ability to conceive.

In more specific terms, Rena's doctor, Dr. Flanders Dunbar, discovered that the muscles surrounding Rena's fallopian tubes—responding to her feelings of fear—would involuntarily contract at the time of ovulation. This tightening of the muscles would close Rena's fallopian tubes during ovulation, thereby preventing her from becoming pregnant. Dr. Dunbar contends that "an emotional crisis or shock may close these tubes just as it may make one clench one's fist."[4] Doctors Howard and Martha Lewis supported Dr. Dunbar's research and concluded that "a woman's emotional problems may make her fallopian tubes involuntarily contract at the time of ovulation—when the egg is produced—making conception impossible."[5]

This study is significant in that it was one of the first I have found that documents how the mind-body connection can directly affect the body's ability to conceive. The contraction of the muscles around the fallopian tubes was precipitated by fear. The body was reacting to an emotional stimulus.

In the past, the medical community has acknowledged psychosomatic disharmonies within the body. It wasn't uncommon for a doctor to conclude that a patient who was under tremendous stress might experience symptoms such as high blood pressure, tension headaches, digestion issues, back spasms, or break out in a skin rash, but infertility was always considered primarily a physiological issue.

In the decades that followed the *Psychosomatics* study, several more studies which investigated the connection between infertility and the emotional well-being of the patient started to surface. One study, conducted at Yale University and published in *Fertility and Sterility* in 1985, looked at the importance of addressing emotional issues that can interfere with conception. The study took a number of women who were trying to get pregnant and split them into two groups: one group worked with a therapist on issues directly related to their infertility while the control group did not receive therapy. Although the study conducted by DeCherney and Sarrel was small, the group that worked with the therapist on issues that were related to their infertility had a 60 percent conception success rate. The control group had an 11 percent pregnancy rate.[6]

In 1993, another study published in *Fertility and Sterility* found that "psychosocial distress contributes significantly to the etiology of some forms of infertility."[7] In simple terms, this study, conducted by Wasser, Sewall, and Soules, concluded that women who were experiencing stress had greater difficulty becoming pregnant. It was not only another validation of how stress and our emotional well-being can affect fertility, but it was one of many studies that began to surface at that time that focused on the mental and emotional components of infertility. The increasing numbers of studies in this area indicated that the scientific community was questioning the traditional belief that infertility was simply a physical phenomenon completely devoid of thought or emotion.

Also in 1993, a study investigated the impact of depression on pregnancy rates. The study, published in *The Journal of Psychosomatic Research*, examined the effects of depression on the success rates of women who were undergoing in vitro (IVF) procedures. The research team called this study "mood state as a predictor of treatment outcome after in vitro fertilization/embryo transfer technology." The women participants were evaluated to determine their "mood state" or level of depression prior to undergoing in vitro procedures. The findings were that women with elevated depression levels had less than half the conception success rates of the women who were not experiencing depression.[8]

The importance of the mood state study was that it showed that depression can be a significant factor in the conception process. Women who are struggling with infertility often report feelings of sadness or hopelessness, feelings of inadequacy or feelings that they are letting down people in their lives. According to Dr. Alice Domar, Director of Women's Health Programs at the Beth Israel Deaconess Medical Center and assistant professor at Harvard Medical School, 30–50 percent of women who experience infertility report "depressive symptoms." When Domar went on to say that the depression and anxiety experienced by women struggling with infertility was equivalent to "women with cancer, HIV status, or heart disease,"[9] it raised some eyebrows. The traditional beliefs—where the fertility process was thought to be removed from all thoughts and emotions—were being challenged.

As with any issue, people have produced studies that argue both sides of the debate about whether there is a connection between the mind and body and a woman's ability to become pregnant. The majority of the research seems to indicate that there is a mind-body relationship when it comes to conception. In the area of infertility, most of the studies have focused on distress and how it affects IVF success rates. This is only one small part of a much larger picture, but it is significant. It is important to note that the methods and diagnostic tools for these studies vary greatly: some have included mind-body programs enabling women to process issues prior to their IVF procedures while others have simply conducted multiple-choice tests to access the degree of distress before IVF procedures have been administered. There have been fourteen major published studies investigating how levels of distress can affect a woman's success when she undergoes an IVF cycle. Dr. Alice Domar summarizes the results of those studies:

> Ten of the studies showed that distress levels are indeed associated with decreased pregnancy rates. The more anxiety or depression the women expressed before undergoing IVF, the less likely they were to get pregnant. In several of the studies, the results were dramatic; for example, in one study the most depressed women experienced half the pregnancy rates of the least depressed women. Two of the fourteen studies had small sample sizes and the results showed trends (i.e. there was a tendency for the distressed women to have lower pregnancy rates), but the re-

sults fell just short of statistical significance. Two of the studies showed no relationship between distress and pregnancy rates.[10]

In the 1990s, studies started to specifically introduce hypnosis as a mind-body modality in an effort to promote conception. The pioneers in this field were Philip Quinn, who was at that time the Director of the Association for Applied Hypnosis, and Dr. Elizabeth Muir. Dr. Muir, a clinical psychologist who now serves as the director of a clinic in London that specializes in working with fertility and childbirth, was a colleague of the late Philip Quinn and gives him credit as the individual who introduced the use of hypnosis as a means of processing the emotional components of infertility. Quinn introduced the term "psychosomatic infertility" because of the connections he observed in which infertility could often be related to psycho-emotional causes. While other people may claim to have been the first to introduce hypnosis as an adjunct to fertility work, I've never found any documentation of studies prior to this one that dealt directly with the use of hypnosis as a method of overcoming infertility. Quinn, along with Dr. Michael Pawson, published the results of their landmark study in 1994, in an article called "Psychosomatic Infertility," published in the *European Journal of Clinical Hypnosis*.[11]

The "Psychosomatic Infertility" study took a group of women between the ages of twenty-six and forty-two (mean of thirty-two years) who had durations of infertility lasting from two to twelve years (with a mean of three and a half years), and each of those women participated in an average of nine hypnotherapy sessions. Nine of those women received additional treatments such as IVF or GIFT (Gamete Intra-Fallopian Transfer) procedures. Twenty-six of the forty women, 65 percent, went on to have successful full-term pregnancies. Quinn and Pawson concluded that:

The inability to make a diagnosis in medically-unexplained infertility and the low success rates in these and other resistant cases tends to indicate that both the cause and to a large extent the

cure in many such instances may lie outside the scope of allopathic medical approaches.[12]

Those words, "the cause and to a large extent the cure in many such instances may lie outside the scope of allopathic medical approaches,"
mean that allopathy, or traditional Western medicine, may not be the
cure or solution to infertility issues.

In addition to the 65 percent success rate in the Quinn and Pawson
study, the successful patients "reported a high incidence of trouble-free
pregnancies, short labors, and uncomplicated births."[13] Almost half of the
women, including women who did not achieve pregnancy, reported an
"alleviation or resolving of various menstrual and gynecological
problems."[14]

While some may argue that the study was too small or that the subjects were too young (with a mean age of thirty-two), the results of this
study were staggering: 65 percent had successful full-term pregnancies,
and these were women who averaged three-and-a-half-year terms of infertility prior to the study. The use of hypnosis as a treatment for infertility in the Quinn and Pawson study generated the highest success rate
of any mind-body research studies, and to the best of my knowledge,
no medical or mind-body research to this day has produced a better live
birth outcome.

Quinn and Pawson drew comparisons between the human condition and behavior in the animal kingdom. "In the wild, situations such
as the loss of a mate, the presence of excessive predators, nest disturbance, overcrowding, migration or unsettled environmental conditions
can cause procreative activity to cease."[15] All of these situations have
counterparts in the human world. For example, a nest disturbance
could mean anything from remodeling to moving or living in a house
or an apartment that is too small to raise a family. The reference to the
presence of a predator may not be an occurrence in the present day: it
may be in the form of a memory of an abusive experience from years
past that has not been adequately processed.

In the conclusion of the study, Quinn and Pawson discussed the advantage of adding hypnosis to a woman's protocol even if she is under-

going medical treatments for infertility: "... limited though this study was, there are still strong indications that both the personal and financial costs of infertility treatments might be considerably reduced by combining a hypnotherapy approach with medical procedures."[16]

Dr. Elizabeth Muir, who worked with Quinn, also observed a connection between emotional issues stored in the subconscious mind and a woman's inability to become pregnant. Muir says that while a woman might consciously want a baby, her subconscious mind may be stopping her from getting pregnant. "Most of the women I see have psychosomatic infertility related to conflicts or unresolved issues about having a baby. A combination of counseling and hypnotherapy can remove these problems."[17] Muir believes that "every thought has an emotional connotation; every emotion has a biochemical counterpart. Therefore, each emotion triggers numerous biochemical changes not only in the brain, but in different parts of the body ..."[18] In other words, our thoughts are constantly affecting our physical biochemistry, the reactions that take place at the cellular level within the physical body. Our thoughts, feeling, and beliefs directly affect what goes on in the physical realm.

Dr. Muir's success rate in working with infertility clients is 45 percent, a number which is based on live births that take place within one year of completing the program she offers at her clinic. That means that 45 percent of these previously infertile women, typically ranging in age from thirty-seven to forty-three, were able not only to conceive, but to give birth. Dr. Muir says—in regard to women who are concerned with the time left on their biological clock—that she believes "psychological and emotional factors, not age, have much more influence on a woman's chances of conceiving."[19]

The success rates of Quinn and Muir generated a great deal of interest. Not only did it show that addressing the mind-body connection was an essential part of promoting conception, but these success rates of 45–65 percent were far better than most fertility specialists had been able to achieve with their most effective and costly assisted reproductive technology (ART): the in vitro procedure. Their research had produced evidence that dealing with the emotional or psychological part of infertility was certainly as important as—and produced better results than—simply addressing the physical issues.

The work of Quinn and Muir inspired more research. A study that introduced a mind-body program to 132 infertility clients, produced a 42 percent success rate (published in the *Journal of the American Medical Women's Association* in 1999). Dr. Alice Domar was one of the three primary facilitators of the study, which was described as a "cognitive-behavioral treatment program" for infertility. Cognitive-behavioral treatment (CBT) can mean any number of processes, including hypnotherapy, in which cognitive therapy (psychotherapy) and behavioral therapy are combined. The objective is that making positive changes in the emotional state (feelings, beliefs, etc.) will generate positive behaviors and outcomes. Dr. Domar found this process to be very beneficial not just in increasing pregnancy rates, but also in helping lessen feelings of depression, anxiety, and anger:

> In four published studies on several hundred women with an infertility duration of 3.5 years, 42 percent conceived within six months of completing the program and there were significant decreases in all measured psychological symptoms including depression, anxiety and anger.[20]

One of the observations made during this study was that the women who had the highest depression scores, at the beginning of the study, went on to have the highest success rates after participating in the mind-body program. The conception success rate for that subset of high depression women in this study was 57 percent.[21]

Another study, also conducted under the supervision of Dr. Alice Domar at the Harvard Medical School and published in *Fertility and Sterility*, involved 184 women who had been trying to conceive for one to two years. The participants were divided into groups: one group took part in a ten-week mind-body program and experienced a 55 percent pregnancy success rate, as opposed a 20 percent conception success rate with the control group. Dr. Domar observed that "in addition, the mind-body patients reported significantly greater psychological improvements."[22]

A study presented at the 2004 European Society of Human Reproduction and Embryology conference in Berlin, by Israeli Professor Eliahu Levitas, M.D., looked at the effects of hypnosis on the success rate for in vitro procedures. The study involved eighty-nine women who experienced hypnosis at the time of embryo transfer and ninety-six women who had transfers without hypnosis. The results showed that 28 percent of the women in the hypnosis group became pregnant as opposed to 14 percent in the control group. Levitas concluded that: "Performing embryo transfer under hypnosis may significantly contribute to an increased clinical pregnancy rate."[23]

It is important to note that the study by Professor Levitas was not designed to process emotional issues that might be at the root of the infertility. It was simply the use of hypnosis to help support women at the time of their transfer, the part of the in vitro procedure where the fertilized eggs are placed back into a woman's uterus. Based on the studies described in this chapter, the evidence indicates that when the mental and emotional issues underlying the infertility are addressed and processed, the success rate is significantly higher than merely adding hypnosis at the time of an IVF transfer.

Processing mental and emotional issues through the use of cognitive-behavioral therapy (CBT) was used in a 2006 study by Professor Sarah Berga, M.D., from Emory University in Atlanta, Georgia, which looked at using CBT in an attempt to restore fertility to women who were suffering from amenorrhea (the inability to ovulate and have periods). Berga found that a woman experiencing excessive stress produced high levels of cortisol, a stress hormone, which in turn inhibits the release of GnRH. GnRH, the gonadotropin-releasing hormone, is the hormone that stimulates ovulation. Dr. Berga found that CBT had a profound effect on the women in the study. She observed "a staggering 80 percent of the women who received CBT started to ovulate again, as opposed to only 25 percent [of the women in the control group]." Follow-up tests indicated that the women who participated in the twenty-week CBT program had lower cortisol levels and higher GnRH levels.[24]

What do all of these numbers mean? There *is* scientific evidence to support the fact that the mind-body connection is of vital importance to the conception process. The numbers from these studies are too significant to ignore, especially when they are compared to the success rates of fertility procedures utilizing traditional Western medicine.

In Western medicine, a woman can choose from a couple of assisted reproductive technologies (ART) to increase her chances of conception. One option is an IUI or intrauterine insemination (see table 2A). In simplest terms, this is when a sample of sperm is artificially inserted into a woman's body. The typical success rate for this procedure is 2–8 percent and the cost is approximately $1,500–$3,000, depending on medications and other variables. Another option is undergoing an IVF or in vitro fertilization procedure (see table 2A) where eggs are harvested from a woman, brought together with sperm in the lab, and then transferred back into the woman's uterus. The success rate for this is higher, approximately 28 percent for younger women, but the cost, often in the range of $12,000 to $25,000, is significantly higher as well.[25] It is important to note that women often undergo multiple attempts when it comes to these procedures. Dr. Randine Lewis, in her book, *The Infertility Cure*, puts these procedures in perspective when she says that most women who choose the Western medical route undergo *seven* ART cycles, spending thousands of dollars in their attempt to get pregnant. [26]

The third option for women is to use a mind-body modality such as hypnosis to strengthen the mind-body connection by reducing the stress response and processing the underlying emotional issues. Based on the studies described above, the success rate of mind-body work falls between 42 and 65 percent and the cost might run anywhere from $500 to $2,000.

If one simply looks at the numbers, the mind-body work makes a powerful statement.

TABLE 2A: INFERTILITY TREATMENTS		
Procedure	Typical Success Rates	Avg. Cost
IUI	2–8%	$1,500–$3,000
IVF	28%	$12,000–$25,000
Mind-body program	42–65%	$500–$2,000

The 28 percent IVF success rate used in Table 2A is based on the findings of the 2004 Assisted Reproductive Technology (ART) Report* from the Center for Disease Control and Prevention, the government agency which tracks this information. In this report, 94,242 women underwent IVF procedures with fresh non-donor eggs, and 28 percent of those women were able to conceive and give birth. Almost half of those women were under age thirty-five. For women over thirty-five, the take-home baby rate was 21 percent, and, for women over forty, the success rate drops into the single digits. It is important to note that the success rates for these medical procedures can depend on variables that range from the age of the woman to medications administered and adjunct procedures used.

Some fertility specialists might to want to challenge the 28 percent success rate for IVF procedures and claim that their numbers are higher, but these are the figures that a woman should use if she is considering this method of ART. The numbers presented by many fertility clinics can be misleading for several reasons. Some clinics count the percentages of pregnancies, even those of very short durations, and present that figure rather than the number of successful pregnancies that result in live births. Some fertility specialists are selective about the types of

---

* It takes several years for the CDC to assimilate the information that goes into an ART report, so there is always a two to three year delay between the last day of the calendar year and the release of the corresponding ART report. This document attempts to record all IVF procedures that were performed in the U.S. over an entire year.

patients with whom they will work. For example, if a woman is too old, her FSH is too high, she has been diagnosed with PCOS, or if there are other limiting factors, a fertility specialist may *discourage* her from undergoing an in vitro procedure by advising her that her chances of success are too low. The other factor that can *significantly* inflate IVF success rates is when doctors *strongly encourage* the use of donor eggs even in cases where that may not be necessary. The patient's chances of achieving pregnancy with donor eggs are much greater, but the trade-off is that the baby does not have a genetic connection to the mother.

These practices make it difficult for a woman to make an accurate comparison of doctors in this field. Women who are considering fertility clinics should ask for figures based on *live births* and *always* ask for the non-donor success rates unless they are specifically interested in a donor cycle. Another important question is to ask about the ratio of women who used donor eggs versus those who used their own eggs at that clinic. This question will clarify if the doctors tend to make recommendations favoring donor eggs.

In looking at these numbers, a woman who is over thirty-five has roughly a one-in-five chance of having a baby if she spends approximately $20,000 on an in vitro procedure. As Dr. Randine Lewis says, most women undergo *seven* ART procedures before they either get pregnant or give up.[26] Assuming a woman has five IUI procedures and two IVF procedures, a fairly common course of action for women using ART, the cost to the couple will likely be in excess of $50,000. In comparison, by doing mind-body work at an average cost of $1,000 for a series of sessions, a woman's chances of conception are two to three times higher than what they would be with an IVF procedure. It makes sense to do the mind-body work first and then consider working with medical drugs and procedures.

The evidence in this chapter indicates that using medical techniques alone for reproduction does not address the entire picture and if the emotional work is ignored, the chance of success can be greatly reduced.

So what is the best approach? For some couples it may be a combination of mind-body work and assisted reproductive technology. Some of the women in the mind-body studies described above simply added hypnosis or some kind of mind-body work to a protocol that included a series of IUIs or an in vitro procedure. The purpose of including the studies in this chapter is not to discourage women from following the medical route, but to make women aware of the mind-body connection and the importance of working on one's mental and emotional issues in order to create a successful pregnancy.

Another option worth consideration is working with a combination of alternative modalities such as hypnotherapy, acupuncture, and Maya uterine massage (see chapter 14) for twelve months before turning to Western medical drugs and procedures. Many women who have explored alternative modalities such as these have found that they were able to conceive without assisted reproductive technology.

Many women admit that they never considered the possibility that their thoughts and emotions might be affecting their fertility. Every day we are learning more and more about the connection between mind and body. It would be shortsighted to believe that our emotions can affect many aspects of our health and yet deny that our thoughts and emotions have anything to do with the process of conception.

So, the question becomes: how can our negative thoughts and emotions affect the ability to conceive? How, exactly, does the mind work? That is the focus of chapter three.

In Their Own Words

The second of the women's stories, Diane's story, is a perfect example of the power of the mind-body connection. Diane was told that she had an elevated FSH of 21 and a low follicle count. Based on traditional medical beliefs regarding infertility, that diagnosis meant that she wouldn't be able to conceive with her own eggs even if she underwent an in vitro procedure. As a result, she was referred to a counselor to deal with her grief.

Rather than accept that her medical diagnosis was the final word, Diane turned to alternative modalities. She learned how to use the mind-body connection to her advantage, and she used that power to reclaim her fertility.

Diane's Story

A Journey from Fear and Infertility to Mind-Body
Awareness and a Healthy Pregnancy

When I was thirty-two, I became pregnant for the first time after about four months of fairly unorganized "trying." I had a healthy pregnancy and typical vaginal birth, using all of the traditional, Western medical strategies for managing labor and delivery.

The years following the birth of my first child were very stressful. I believe I suffered from some postpartum depression until my baby was about nine months old, but I was never diagnosed or treated for it. My job was very stressful and I went back to work after about six weeks. I struggled constantly with childcare and the associated feelings of guilt and resentment about having to juggle so much.

By the time my daughter was three years old, I had had enough, and I decided to leave my job. This was a very traumatic transition that took a very long time to complete. I did not have very good support from friends, family, or child care providers during this time, and I often felt isolated and lonely as a parent.

Once my daughter started preschool and I left my job, I found many new friends through her school. This was a very important experience for me and gave me a new sense of my identity as a mother and as a woman. I felt validated in these new roles for the first time. As a result, I felt strong enough and secure enough in my new understanding of and new-found joy in being a mother, that my husband and I decided we were ready for another baby.

We started trying to conceive in January 2003 and by July I still was not pregnant. I had also been suffering from a really serious bout of bronchitis and the flu, and just could not seem to get well. I was feeling depressed about being sick and about not getting pregnant. I also had a very strong, intuitive sense that something was not right with my body and with my reproductive health. During this time, I was seeing my primary-care doctor fairly often because of my bronchitis and because I was having a hard time getting healthy; I was diagnosed with hypothyroidism during this time as well. My primary-care doctor thought the hypothyroidism might be the reason I was having trouble getting pregnant, but she referred me to a reproductive endocrinologist anyway.

I visited the reproductive endocrinologist in July 2003 and received a diagnosis of an elevated FSH of 21 and a very low follicle count. The doctor told me I was not a good candidate for any of the technical strategies they could offer. Instead, I was referred to a counselor to deal with the grief and confusion of infertility, and to an acupuncturist/Chinese medicine practitioner specializing in treating infertility.

I don't think I had known anything about the mind-body connection before I met my acupuncturist or my hypnotherapist. I started seeing my acupuncturist with an attitude of "I have nothing to lose" now that I am officially infertile and unable to conceive, but she changed my whole perspective on health right away. She explained to me that "harder, stronger, faster, longer" is not necessarily a healthy way to approach exercise and life in general and represents a very Western mindset. She also helped me to understand the very serious impact stress can have on overall health, and reproductive health in particular. She gave me many books and articles to read, recommended nutrition and exercise strategies, and introduced me to restorative yoga. I took Chinese herbs and did everything she told me to do. I really changed my life in some very profound and lasting ways, and my body was feeling better than it had ever felt, at a very deep, cellular level. However, I hadn't yet changed my mind.

I had one very serious block, and that was the diagnosis I had received from the reproductive endocrinologist: an FSH of 21 means you can't get pregnant, you're halfway to menopause and you're infertile. So, as much as my acupuncturist believed that I could get pregnant, and as much as I believed in everything she was doing, I didn't actually believe that any of it was going to help get me pregnant. When I talked to her about this, she referred me to a hypnotherapist.

My hypnotherapist was the one who really educated me about what the mind-body connection means and how much influence my subconscious was having on my physical reproductive health. I worked with hypnosis to specifically overcome the conscious block that was impeding my full reproductive health. This block was a mental barrier, and no matter how ready my body might be for a pregnancy, my mind had decided that the FSH diagnosis was the final word. Working with mind-body techniques, I developed a very compassionate and profound sense of my mind's role in my journey toward fertility. The work in hypnosis helped me develop many positive visualizations, with meditation and relaxation techniques, and most importantly, with a conscious mantra to affirm my strength and fertility: "I am strong, healthy and fertile." I would meditate on this while doing yoga, during acupuncture treatments and massages, and while just driving in the car or lying in bed. It helped me immensely because I believe that this experience with hypnotherapy, and being educated in the mind-body connection by my practitioners, enabled me to make a complete connection between my mind and my body which led me to become pregnant *naturally* with a son. This process led me to re-think my entire perspective on what it means to be *well*. When I look back, prior to mind-body work, I realize how disjointed my life and my self-awareness was. Since this experience, I now feel integrated and whole for the first time in my life, and the addition of our son [to our family] has brought much happiness in our lives.

WORKS CITED

1. Lewis, Howard R. and Martha E. Lewis. *Psychosomatics* (New York, New York: Pinnacle Books, 1972).
2. Ibid., 210–211.
3. Ibid., 211.

4. Ibid., 210.

5. Ibid., 210.

6. Sarrel, and A. DeCherney, *Fertility and Sterility* 43 (1985): 897–000.

7. S. Wasser, G. Sewall, and M. Soules. "Psychosocial stress as a cause of infertility," *Fertility and Sterility* 59 (1993): 685–689.

8. P. Thiering, J. Beaurepaire, M. Jones, et al., "Mood state as a predictor of treatment outcome after in vitro fertilization/embryo transfer technology (IVT/ET)," *Journal of Psychosomatic Research* 37 (1993): 481–491.

9. Alice D. Domar, *The Journal of Psychosomatic Obstetrics and Gynecology* 14, Suppl. (1993): 45–52.

10. Domar, Alice D., "Infertility and Stress," *www.bostonivf.com/mind_body_center/InfertilityandStress.pdf*, 1–5.

11. Philip Quinn DR, and Michael Pawson MB BS FRCOG. "Psychosomatic Infertility," *European Journal of Clinical Hypnosis* Volume 4 (July 1994): 1–10.

12. Ibid., 3.

13. Ibid., 1.

14. Ibid., 1.

15. Ibid., 3.

16. Ibid., 10.

17. Louise Manson, "Baby talk," *Sunday Times*, July 19, 1998.

18. Jim Schwartz, BCH, "The mind-body approach to fertility, An Interview with Dr. Elizabeth Muir," *Resolve Newsletter* (Winter 2004): 10–11.

19. Manson, "Baby Talk."

20. A. D. Domar, P. C. Zuttermeister, M. Seibel, and H. Benson, "Psychological improvement in infertile women after behavioral treatment: a replication." *Fertility and Sterility*, 58 (1992): 144–147.

21. A. D. Domar, and H. Dreher. *Healing Mind, Healthy Woman* (Diane Publishing Co., 1996): 238.

22. A. D. Domar, et al. "Impact of group psychological interventions on pregnancy rates in infertile women." *Fertility and Sterility*, 73 (2000): 805–811.

23. David Brinn, "Israeli study proves hypnosis can double IVF success rate." Our Jerusalem, http://www.ourjerusalem.com/news/story/news2004 0824.html, August 22, 2004.

24. Kathy Jones, "Behavioral therapy helps stress-induced infertility" http://www.foodconsumer.org/cgi-bin/777/exec/view.cgi/20/3939/printer, June 21, 2006.

25. Numbers based on reports from SART and the 2004 ART Report from the Center for Disease Control and Prevention. http://www.cdc.gov/ART/ART2004/section2a.htm#11.

26. Randine Lewis, *The Infertility Cure* (New York: Little, Brown and Company, 2004), 5.

CHAPTER THREE

HOW THE MIND WORKS

The evidence presented in chapter two indicates that the mind-body connection is vitally important to the conception process. Our emotions, fears, and beliefs, which lie hidden in our psyche, create stress and play a significant role in reproduction. In order to get a clear understanding of these dynamics, it is important to examine how the mind works.

AN OVERVIEW

Inside our brains, we have a conscious and a subconscious mind (see figure 3.1, page 39). The conscious mind, often referred to as the critical mind, is the part of the brain that is logical and analytical. It does the reasoning. It is the part of the mind that keeps us functioning throughout the day and the part that is utilized as we make most of our daily decisions. When we do things like work on the computer or pay bills, we are working with the conscious or critical mind. Much of our day is spent doing tasks that involve the conscious or critical mind.

On the other hand, the subconscious mind stores our habits, beliefs, behavioral patterns, anxieties, and fears. It is the part of our mind that makes us feel and experience emotions. When we experience things like frustration, anger, sadness, or fear; when we become overwhelmed by stress; when we demonstrate compulsive behavior like perfectionism; or when we have an insatiable craving for food or sweets, we are responding to the information or programming of the subconscious mind. All significant emotional issues of our past are stored here and dictate how we feel and how we emotionally react to current-day events and challenges. For example, a trip to the doctor that frightened and traumatized us at age two—which our *conscious* mind may no longer remember—may still cause us to be abnormally anxious and fearful of medical care. The subconscious mind has recorded this initiating event and that event can become a source of the mysterious anxiety and fear that affects us each time we visit the physician. Until that memory is identified and addressed, the uneasiness related to medical care and doctors will remain in place. All of our life issues are stored in the subconscious mind, and in order to make genuine and lasting changes, those changes and the healing must take place at the subconscious level.

The reason it is difficult to recall or identify buried memories, such as the visit to the doctor's office at age two, is due to a protective wall or barrier surrounding the subconscious mind called the *critical factor* (see figure 3.1). One of the functions of the critical factor is to protect us from having to relive painful emotions and experiences of our past, but at the same time it is concealing valuable information that is at the root of much of our behavior. That memory from age two is buried because of the critical factor: we don't remember the specifics of that doctor's visit in our conscious mind, but the emotional charge from that experience continues to generate uneasiness. The end result is that we experience anxiety when we seek medical attention, but we have no conscious information as to the origin of the uncomfortable reaction.

How does this relate to infertility? The source of our stress and the emotional blocks to fertility often lie deeply concealed in the subconscious mind. In order to uncover this material, we have to find a way around the critical factor, that wall that keeps us from consciously knowing the root of the problem. Interestingly enough, most of the issues that block fertility aren't huge traumatic events. Oftentimes it is simple subconscious programming such as feelings of inadequacy that interfere with conception.

Here is a more in-depth look at how the mind works and how hidden issues can affect fertility.

THE SUBCONSCIOUS MIND

Most people don't realize or appreciate the incredible power of the sub-conscious mind. In a subtle way, it is controlling most of our everyday emotions and behaviors. When someone feels anxious, is compulsive about cleaning, needs to have a cigarette, or beats themselves up for a mistake that they've made, they are following the information written in their subconscious programming.

In a way, it is very similar to how a computer works. Our subconscious minds have been programmed by every event that has occurred in our lifetime. Some of the most powerful programming takes place when we are very young, especially during the first five years of life. This programming remains in place in our adult life. It affects our emotions and behaviors until we identify the source and process the underlying issues.

An easy way to understand how our subconscious programming works is to look at a hypothetical example. Imagine someone who is programmed for emotional eating. Every time that person is hurt or upset, they turn to food—often sweets—in an attempt to make themselves feel better. Their body might feel full, but there is something that pushes them to continue eating.

How would a pattern like this begin? Imagine that emotional eater as a five-year-old child coming home after school and crying to her mother because she had been bullied on the playground. To make that child feel better, mom produces a plate of chocolate chip cookies accompanied by words like "it'll be okay." A month later, when that child falls and skins her knees, her parents give her a big bowl of ice cream with the assurance that "this will make you feel better." A pattern begins to develop, and each time food or sweets are used to help calm the emotional response the reinforcement becomes stronger. The programming that goes into this child's subconscious mind is that if she becomes sad or angry or hurt, she should turn to comfort foods to make her feel better. Then, after that child becomes an adult, whenever there is an emotional upset—such as an argument with her husband, a conflict at work or a criticism that hurts her feelings—she instinctively starts eating, usually with no knowledge of the subconscious programming that is driving her behavior.

That response has been "programmed" into the subconscious mind. That person might try to go on a diet, but as soon as she feels sad, lonely, angry, hurt, or any one of a number of negative emotions that might be stored in her memory, the trigger in the subconscious mind is engaged and the emotional eater will return to the old habits.

What this means is that *one has to change the programming in the subconscious mind if one wants to change the corresponding behavior.* If we don't deal with the programming, then the trigger that is driving the behavior—in this case, the emotional eating—is still in place.

The way the programming is changed is by addressing the subconscious emotions and issues that provide the basis or foundation on which the programming has been built. It all starts with resolving the source material that is driving our thoughts, beliefs, and emotions. To correct the habits of that emotional eater, the underlying issues or source information must be addressed, and only then will the programming change. This is why diets and dietary regimens are rarely successful. Unless the client is also actively working to heal the wound or belief system that is at the root of the programming, the old behavior and habits never go away.

So, the subconscious mind records all of the events and emotions from our past and that, in turn, influences our behavior and decisions we make today.

How does this apply to one's ability to conceive? Many of the issues that are recorded or programmed into the subconscious mind—such as feelings of inadequacy, concerns about body image, perfectionism, dysfunctional family relationships, miscarriages, fear of childbirth, abortions, and childhood abuse—are blocks to conception. Our ability to conceive is directly related to our emotional well-being and it often necessitates processing and healing of emotional issues in order for conception to take place. I've witnessed this phenomenon in my practice for years, and with more and more scientific studies to support the mind-body connection and its relationship to fertility we are beginning to understand why so many cases are being labeled as "unexplained." (The research studies in chapter two document the benefits of healing the subconscious in order to promote fertility.) Negative beliefs and emotions can generate feelings such as guilt, shame, inadequacy, anxiety, and fear, all of which can be powerful enough to prevent conception.

HOW FEELINGS AND EMOTIONS
ARE OFTEN MISTAKEN FOR STRESS

As negative feelings manifest in the body, they are often carelessly generalized into the catch-all category of "stress." It is true that all of these feelings create stress in our bodies, but by generalizing these emotions into one category, it often becomes very easy to misdiagnose the true source of the emotional material. When most people hear the word "stress" they automatically think of things like being overwhelmed at work or having too much to do around the house, or situations such as having to take care of an ailing family member. While those types of things do create stress and do impact the ability to conceive, that catch-all word of stress causes us to overlook some of the root issues that are really blocking the fertility. Work stress may be misidentified as the cause of a woman's infertility while the true source may be fear or guilt or a number of other emotions whose true roots come from earlier life experiences or traumas. These old issues, lodged in the subconscious mind, are the true source of the stress while the conditions at the workplace are simply enhancing or multiplying the condition.

To understand this misdiagnosis, it helps to take a hypothetical example: a woman who has had an abortion. Most women who have had an abortion feel tremendous guilt. Left unprocessed, this guilt stays with them for the rest of their lives. Women often believe that the reason they are experiencing infertility is because of the termination. As a form of self-punishment, it isn't uncommon for a woman who has had an abortion to make a subconscious decision that she will never forgive herself. This guilt creates incredible stress. When she sees an infertility specialist, the doctor might tell this patient that she needs to relax and reduce her stress level. Immediately, when the patient hears the word stress, she assumes that it must be work-related, and she needs to cut back on her hours at work. While it is true that work stress can be a factor in infertility, the major stress that this woman is experiencing is more likely due to her guilt and feeling unforgiven for the abortion. The negative emotions and issues from our past that are generated from the subconscious mind create what we have come to collectively label as stress, and we feel this stress every day until we process and heal the source of it. It is essential to understand that stress has everything to do with old feelings, emotions, and issues, and our daily workload is simply compounding what we have been holding inside all of our lives. Therefore, the stress diagnosis is often misunderstood: cutting back at work is only a small part of a much larger picture.

How can stress or negative feelings and emotions affect the body on a physical level? It can cause many reproductive disharmonies including:

- Inadequate uterine blood flow.
- Poor follicle production and quality.
- Increased cortisol levels, which inhibits the release of GnRH, the gonadotropin-releasing hormone, which is the hormone that stimulates ovulation. Increased cortisol can also block progesterone receptors, which, in turn, can create difficulties with embryo implantation.
- Creation of a negative response by the hypothalamus gland, the gland which is considered to be the control center in the brain for reproductive activity. (See chapter four for more information about the stress response and the hypothalamus gland.) The hypothalamus can essentially switch off reproductive functions (including balanced hormone production) when it is stressed.
- Weakening of the adrenal glands, which can lead to the lowering of progesterone levels.
- The triggering of the fight-or-flight response where the blood moves to the extremities and away from the reproductive organs. This is accompanied by the engaging of the sympathetic nervous system which is the placement of the body into the stress mode. Symptoms of this response might include an elevated heart rate, higher blood pressure, and constricted blood vessels.

- Disruption of the function of the pituitary gland's production of hormones. This can adversely affect the hormones responsible for ovulation and regular menstruation.
- Creation of uterine fibroids.
- Irregular cycles.
- Increased prolactin levels, which can interfere with ovulation.

This list is certainly not comprehensive as there are other adverse effects that stress can have on our ability to reproduce; however, many of the conditions on this list are enough on their own to cause infertility. It is also important to note that *the conditions on this list are sometimes used to explain infertility as having a physiological cause or root when the true issue might be the emotional stress that is creating these disharmonies.*

Some people might argue that the emotions can't affect our physical bodies, or they might believe in certain psychosomatic disharmonies but not believe in psychosomatic infertility. It is time to look at this belief from a different point of view. If millions of women around the world have been diagnosed with unexplained infertility, we have no choice but to explore the mental/emotional realm. And how do we heal the emotional roots? We have to work with what has been programmed within the subconscious mind. To understand how our thoughts and emotions affect us, it is important to get an understanding of the dynamics between the subconscious mind, the conscious mind, and the critical factor.

THE CONSCIOUS MIND

What role does the conscious or critical mind play in the overall infertility picture? The conscious mind is for the most part going to be cooperative in the conception process because it is the thinking part of the brain. It is our conscious mind that decides that the time is right to get pregnant and start a family. For example, the conscious mind of a woman with infertility might say: "Now that I've worked my way up the corporate ladder and have become a director in the company, I'm ready to have a baby." In other words, I've completed Step A and now it is time for Step B. Very logical, and a perfect example of critical mind thinking.

But what is going on within the subconscious mind of that woman? It is likely to be saying something like, "You work fifty to sixty hours a week. You don't have any time for a baby. Your body is tired and doesn't have the chi, or energy, to produce and carry a baby. Your workload is never going to get any easier. You have to choose: either you can stay with this career for which you've worked so hard, or you can have a baby. You can't do both." Until there is some reconciliation between the conscious and subconscious minds, this career woman will probably remain enmeshed in her career and not be able to experience motherhood. That doesn't mean that career women need to quit their jobs in order to conceive. It does mean that the subconscious programming needs to be addressed, and ideally a compromise or solution can be reached. If the subconscious material is ignored, then nothing changes. That is why healers often use the phrase: "if nothing changes, nothing changes."

THE CRITICAL FACTOR

We've already established that when you decide you want to make significant changes in your life—habits, lifestyle, beliefs, fears, behavioral patterns—those changes have to be made at the subconscious level. However, making those changes is not an easy process because it involves getting around the critical factor, a formidable line of resistance (see figure 3.1). The job of the critical factor is to try to keep us from being exposed to those negative feelings and emotions within the subconscious. After all, we don't want an overwhelming feeling of sadness to come on in the middle of a business meeting. Under normal circumstances, the critical factor keeps us separated from those negative feelings and memories within the subconscious. In other words, the things we need to heal most are protected by a heavily guarded fortress.

Sometimes it is easier to understand the critical factor if we look at it as a denial wall. The critical factor is much more complex than simply a denial wall, but it might help to think of it that way in order to explain its function.

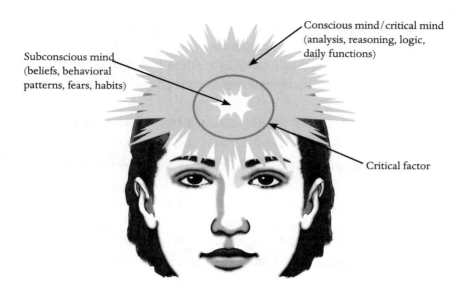

Subconscious mind
(beliefs, behavioral
patterns, fears, habits)

Conscious mind/critical mind
(analysis, reasoning, logic,
daily functions)

Critical factor

Figure 3.1: The subconscious and conscious minds and critical factor.

The person with a steadfast denial wall always pretends that everything is fine. If you say something to them like, "I understand that you had a difficult childhood," they might respond with, "Oh, that's all behind me now," "I learned how to take care of myself at an early age, so it wasn't all bad," or even "What are you talking about?" That person has so much denial that the critical factor—or wall of resistance around the subconscious mind—is large and secure and certainly not about to expose any negative emotions.

Some people—especially those in denial—feel that if we stay protected from our subconscious minds, then we can ignore the issues that are lurking inside and attempt to function without any upsets in our lives. This works better for some individuals than others because those subconscious issues that we often try to suppress have a sneaky way of creeping into our daily life. People who are anxious, fearful, controlling, depressed, feeling inadequate, weepy, or people who have explosive tempers may be trying to suppress what is held inside the subconscious, but those memories and emotions are still seeping out and affecting them every single day. In other words, we may try to pretend that everything is okay and ignore our subconscious material, but it is actually a very powerful force that is continually controlling many of our feelings, behaviors, and even our physical well-being.

HOW TO BYPASS THE CRITICAL FACTOR AND WORK
WITH THE SUBCONSCIOUS MIND

How does one bypass the critical factor and gain access to the subconscious mind? That takes a determined effort because the critical factor can be a powerful fortress. Can it be done by talking to an empathetic friend or sharing your thoughts with a support group? These are valuable processes, and while sharing with people who care is very nurturing, the critical factor doesn't often let its guard down in normal conversations. It is extremely unlikely that ordinary dialogue is going to bypass the critical factor and make its way to the subconscious level where the healing needs to take place. One indication of this is that when deep subconscious healing occurs, it almost always involves:

1. An emotional release.
2. An awakening or new understanding of the issue. There is a breakthrough or discovery where the issue can be looked at objectively and now has a completely different meaning.
3. Profound healing and processing work. Naturally, this step requires the assistance of a skilled practitioner. When this step is complete, the issue no longer carries the same degree of weight. In other words, the client can look at that concern—that used to feel so overwhelming—with a sense of resolution.

There is nothing subtle about this process. When one undergoes all of these experiences, they are *very aware* that a major shift has occurred. True subconscious healing is powerful. At the end of the session, the client may feel somewhat drained, like an enormous weight has been lifted and what was once an overwhelming issue has been released.

Can this work be done in talk therapy? Talk therapy is very beneficial, and the support of a counselor can be a valuable part of the healing process. If, during the therapy session, the client goes through the experience described above, then it is likely that they are working with the subconscious material and making changes that will last a lifetime. Again, this is a powerful process, and the client will have no doubt when they leave the office that a major change or shift has taken place.

However, clients often report that this level of reaction is not a common occurrence in counseling sessions. When the talk therapy involves ordinary conversations where straightforward discussions of the issues take place, that type of work is primarily engaging the *conscious* mind, and the conscious mind is very skilled at protecting our vulnerability. In conventional talk therapy, the client will usually bump up against the critical factor and rarely be able to get to the deep issues buried within the subconscious mind. That isn't to say that this type of psychotherapy isn't beneficial: it can be extremely beneficial. However, the reality is that bypassing the critical factor is not likely to take place under those conditions and therefore that is not an efficient or expeditious way to access what is buried in the subconscious mind. It is important to note that sometimes clients aren't ready or able to do the deep work, and in those cases, conventional talk therapy is an ideal support system. In other words, there are many situations where talk therapy is exactly what a client needs, but if the objective is to access and process the subconscious programming, it is unlikely to happen in ordinary conversation.

What about prayer? Prayer has many benefits and is very important in shaping lives and behavior. The positive attributes of prayer are far-reaching, and the act of praying has given strength to people the world over. Studies have proven the power of prayer as an adjunct to the healing process. It is impossible to even begin to describe the value of prayer in this world. It is important to understand, however, that traditional prayer work is a *conscious* process, and traditional prayer work is *not* designed to bypass the critical factor and access the subconscious material. If prayers were designed to target the subconscious issues, the objective of the prayer would be to ask for the hurt or pain or emotions to emerge and bring the conflicts or issues to the surface where they can be dealt with directly. In other words, the prayer would essentially be saying: "bring up all of my issues and emotions so I can process them, and don't hold anything back." I have never come across any form of traditional prayer work that uses this approach. Without the guidance of some kind of practitioner or healer, that experience could be devastating and potentially very damaging. People should be cautioned to never try that type of processing work on their own and understand that this example was included here simply to illustrate a point about how the subconscious mind is not accessed in traditional prayer work.

There is an exception to the use of prayer work and tapping into the subconscious mind. If the prayer occurs in a very deep trance state, such as what a Buddhist monk might experience, then it is possible to work with the subconscious mind under those circumstances. Again, while the information might be available in that profound state of trance, it is essential to work with a professional who has experience in processing the issues that surface. It is not advisable to try doing this work on your own.

It is important to clarify the information here. Prayer work, traditional talk therapy and working with support groups are all very valuable and important ways of facilitating the healing process. However, these modalities are *not designed to bypass the critical factor* and access subconscious material. That isn't the goal or objective of these processes. It isn't that these modalities aren't beneficial; it is simply being stated that these therapies aren't designed to do deep work at the subconscious level. That is why some people report that they still feel stuck after years of working on their stuff—all of the work they have done may have been at the conscious level, and the subconscious mind was never engaged. It is important to make this distinction because *a woman who wants to address the emotional material that is blocking conception needs to include a healing modality that works directly with her subconscious material if she wants to open the door to conception.*

The safest and most effective way to bypass the critical factor and work directly with the subconscious mind is through the use of hypnotherapy. That is exactly what hypnosis is designed to do, and the fact that hypnosis has been practiced for thousands of years is a testament to its efficacy. This is why so many psychotherapists are now including hypnosis as one of their healing modalities.

WHAT IS HYPNOTHERAPY
AND HOW DOES IT WORK?

Hypnosis is a process where a client enters what is called a "trance state," where they can work directly with the information within the subconscious mind without interference from the critical factor or critical mind. Since the subconscious mind is the source of all of our beliefs, fears, anxieties, emotions, behaviors, and habits, that is where the work needs to be done to create positive changes in our lives. In hypnosis, the root of a problem or block can be identified, and the negative programming associated with that issue can be replaced with positive ideas and suggestions, clearing the way for dramatic life changes. The process is safe, and the benefits can last a lifetime.

There are many misconceptions about hypnosis because of the way it has been portrayed in the movies. It is important to clear up those fallacies. In the movies, there is often a mad scientist who is controlling the behavior of his subjects and having them do activities such as robbing banks. Nothing could be further from the truth. In fact, one of the first things all hypnotists are taught is that "all hypnosis is self-hypnosis." In other words, *the client is in control one hundred percent of the time*, not the hypnotist. Any beliefs that hypnosis is mind-control are completely unfounded. If mind-control were possible through hypnosis, there would be thousands of incidents throughout history, and in the present day, where unscrupulous individuals would have used hypnosis for their own personal gain. There are none. It is impossible because the client is in control, not the hypnotist.

Another misconception is that the client will come out of trance and not remember anything that went on in the session. This is a common occurrence in movies where the hypnotist instructs the subject to do something like rob banks, bring the money back to the hypnotist and then forget everything. Naturally, if the subject remembered anything that happened while they were working with the hypnotist, they could easily identify the true culprit and the movie would be over. They have to forget everything or else the writers have no story. That's how it works in the movies; *in real life, clients remember all that goes on in a session.* How could a client learn how to use techniques such as visualization if they can't remember anything when the session is over?

There is also the truth serum fallacy: the belief that the client will reveal all of their deep dark secrets while they are in trace. Again, the client is in control the entire time. They have the ability to decide what information they want to share or don't want to share.

And what about those actors in the movies who get stuck in trance? If that were a possibility, the government would make it illegal to practice hypnotherapy. Only movie actors get stuck in trance. In my years of research, I've never come across a case where a client became stuck in trance.

The popular notion that people are asleep in hypnosis is yet another movie myth. Although it is very dramatic when the mad scientist is able to utter those classic words: "Go to sleep," the truth is, people *do not* sleep in hypnosis. If a client slept through a hypnosis session, they would get nothing out of it. It is similar to when a person falls asleep while watching a movie: how much of that movie can be recalled the next day? How could a client work on subconscious issues if they were asleep? There has to be interaction, such as discussion, between the hypnotist and the client or else it would be much like sleeping through a psychotherapy session. Hypnosis has nothing to do with sleeping *except* when it is dramatized in the movies.

What is the experience like? Hypnosis occurs naturally and often in daily life. An example of this is when we watch a very engrossing movie and find ourselves emotionally involved. In a sense, being absorbed in that movie is just like being in a trance. Something in that movie is connecting with or engaging the information in the subconscious mind—exactly what happens in hypnosis—and that is why it elicits an emotional reaction. And since being wrapped up in a movie is a form of hypnosis or trance state, we can check in with the movie misconceptions about hypnosis and see if any of them are true. When you are engaged in that movie are you asleep? No. Are you going to rob a bank if the person sitting behind you asks you to do so? No. Are you going to turn to the person in the next seat and tell them your deepest, darkest secrets? No. Do you immediately forget everything that happened in the movie as soon as the credits start to roll? No. If someone told you the theater was on fire and you needed to leave, would you be able to do so, or are you out of control? You could leave. So, we have all entered hypnosis and various trance states, and we do it fairly often.

Hypnosis is very similar to meditation or using one's imagination. The hypnotist uses what is called an induction to help the client—who, again, is always the one in control—enter hypnosis. At that point, there is often interaction where the hypnotherapist and the client will discuss things that are relevant to what that client wants to achieve. The hypnotherapist might ask the client to imagine an experience or emotion related to the current issue in order to elicit a response from the subconscious mind. When that issue comes to the surface, the hypnotherapist will work with the client by guiding them through the act of processing and healing the source of the issue. At the end of the session, the hypnotist will guide the client out of the relaxed state into present awareness.

Naturally, this is a very simplified version of what goes on in a session, but the goal here is to demystify the process to show that hypnotherapy is a safe process. (There is a more detailed explanation of hypnotherapy in the Complementary Modalities chapter.) This new understanding will hopefully remove any of the fears and misconceptions associated with this practice. It is the only healing modality designed to work specifically with the subconscious mind, so it is important that people who want to make life changes—whether it be associated with infertility or not—be comfortable with the process and have an understanding of how it works.

HOW POWERFUL ARE THE ISSUES
IN THE SUBCONSCIOUS MIND?

The power of the subconscious mind has been greatly underestimated. Recent research using powerful neuroimaging technology indicates that the subconscious mind might be the driving force in our lives 95 percent of the time, while the conscious mind affects only about 5 percent of our cognitive activity.[1] An article published in the *U.S. News and World Report* says that "According to cognitive neuroscientists, we are conscious of only about 5 percent of our cognitive activity, so most of our decisions, actions, emotions, and behavior depend on the 95 percent of brain activity that goes beyond our conscious awareness."[2] Most people, if asked whether the conscious mind or the subconscious mind is in charge, probably would have insisted it is the conscious mind. Furthermore, prior to this new research, many people would have guessed that those numbers had accidentally been reversed.

This new information has serious implications. *If the subconscious mind is controlling 95 percent of our cognitive activity, then it becomes even more important to take inventory of the subconscious material.* The woman who has several unprocessed issues may be in a situation where 5 percent of her mind is saying "I want a baby," while the other 95 percent might be working against her. Since our bodies respond to the messages we send (see chapter eight about cellular reprogramming), every thought or feeling becomes a signal that goes directly to the programming of our cells.

CONCLUSION

It is my belief, based on the work that I do and the numerous studies outlined in chapter two, that many women have unprocessed emotional issues that are blocking their ability to conceive and only when they identify and process these issues will they be able to become pregnant. These issues are deeply ingrained in the subconscious mind and that is where the healing must take place. The critical factor or barrier that protects the programming within the subconscious mind has to be bypassed or overcome in order to do this type of work.

Deep trance meditation, highly emotional psychotherapy, and hypnosis are methods of bypassing the critical factor and working directly with subconscious material. Hypnotherapy is one of the few modalities specifically designed to do this kind of work.

It is very important for a client to be working with someone who can guide them through the healing. I often hear clients say, "I thought I could heal that all by myself." That is similar to what Benjamin Franklin said about being your own legal counsel: "A man who is his own lawyer has a fool for a client." The same is true for trying to be your own healer. If you think about it realistically, how could someone possibly look at the issues and experiences that have affected their life so profoundly, be completely objective about those issues, and know exactly what is needed for healing and processing to occur. If it was that simple, then we could easily heal all of our past issues and we wouldn't need therapists or healers. If we had that innate information and ability, then those events and experiences would never have become issues and stayed with us all these years. That doesn't mean that once we hire a therapist we should *expect* them to heal us. We have to take responsibility for our own healing. And, as we do this work and heal the subconscious material, the wonderful part of it is that our lives transform and evolve in very positive ways.

In Their Own Words

The story selected for inclusion in this chapter, Monica's story, again presents a contrast between a holistic approach to fertility and working with assisted reproductive techniques. Many women start their journey by working with Western medical practitioners and then change their focus because they want a more natural course of action. I believe that women should begin with the holistic approach and then, if necessary, pursue medical options.

Monica suspected that the block to her fertility might be hidden in the mental/emotional realm, an area that wasn't being addressed with traditional medicine. Her story illustrates how critical it was to unearth and heal the information in her subconscious mind.

Monica's Story
Beating the Odds

My husband and I married in August 2000, when I was thirty-four. I stopped using birth control pills and became pregnant a couple of months later. Unfortunately that pregnancy ended in a miscarriage that was not discovered until my first ultrasound at ten weeks. Since we had gotten pregnant so quickly I did not imagine that we would have any problem when we tried again. We waited another six months before actively trying again. When another six months went by and I was still not pregnant, I decided to have some tests done.

I went to a well-respected fertility clinic and was diagnosed with high FSH (follicle-stimulating hormone) in January 2003, a couple of months before I turned thirty-seven. I was told by the fertility specialist that I had only a 0–5 percent chance of conceiving with my own eggs and that IVF (in vitro fertilization) would be a waste of time because my eggs were likely to be of such low quality that they would be too fragile to make spending the money on the process worthwhile. The doctors suggested my best bet would be to have IVF with donor eggs.

After receiving this diagnosis, I did as many IUIs (intrauterine inseminations) as they would allow me to do; one with the fertility medication, Clomid; several with Letrazole; and one with injectibles (Repronex), to see how I would respond (the thought being that if I produced a lot of follicles maybe it would be worth trying IVF). I had a few months where I had to rest because I had leftover cysts that prevented treatment that month.

After nine months of physically feeling worse than I ever had in my life, taking the drugs (with side effects of weight gain and mood swings), and after responding terribly to the injectibles (fewer follicles than with the Letrazole), I decided to go in the completely opposite direction and try alternative therapies exclusively.

In addition to acupuncture and Chinese herbs that I had started when I first got the high FSH diagnosis, I began a series of hypnotherapy sessions. I thought maybe there was a subconscious fear or issue that I did not consciously recognize that was preventing me from getting pregnant.

Hypnotherapy was beneficial to me because it was supremely relaxing and it helped me focus my mind in a positive direction with respect to fertility. So much of what I had heard up to that point was negative, about my body and about my fertility. I physically felt like a failure. I felt like my body had betrayed me, and I felt so hopeless. Hypnotherapy helped me to replace those negative thoughts and images with positive, nurturing, encouraging, hopeful, and happy thoughts and images. I stopped focusing on what my body was *not* doing and instead focused on what it *was* doing, what it *could* do, and how very special it was.

During my hypnotherapy sessions that were focused on fertility, some emotional issues involving my family came up. These were, of course, things that I had dealt with in talk therapy over the years and were not anything all that new, but they did seem to be getting in the way of my positive path. So I spent a few extra sessions just on those issues.

It was amazing to me how helpful those sessions were. Issues I had spent years on just *felt* better than they ever had before. There is a saying that goes like this: "talk therapy is like pruning a bush, clipping the branches and keeping it under control, but hypnotherapy is like pulling the bush out roots and all." And that's how I felt—like I really got to the root of the problem and resolved it in a way I had never been able to in a traditional counseling session.

I have no idea if addressing those, what I considered to be *side* emotional issues, had anything to do with promoting my fertility, but it was certainly helpful to my general well-being. And I figured being happier and feeling better about myself could only have a positive effect.

Ultimately I did get pregnant naturally, without any drugs. Not just once, but twice I beat the "0–5 percent chance" I had been given by a fertility specialist. In January 2005, at age thirty-eight, I had my first beautiful daughter, and in May 2006, at age forty, I had another beautiful daughter. I am still amazed every day at the miracle of their presence.

WORKS CITED

1. Marianne Szegedy-Maszak, "Mysteries of the Mind: Your unconscious is making your everyday decisions," *U.S. News and World Report* (Feb. 28, 2005).

2. Ibid.

CHAPTER FOUR

THE STRESS RESPONSE
AND THE IMPORTANCE
OF STRESS REDUCTION

STRESS COMES FROM OUR ISSUES

As discussed in the previous chapter, many people consider stress to be the outcome of what is going on in their present and immediate environment. They look no further than the day-to-day concerns—their job, paying the bills, upkeep on the house, conflicts with their spouse or relatives—and overlook the issues that are often the true source of stress. Issues from the past such as abortions, miscarriages, perfectionism, fear of failure, and feelings of inadequacy can often be generating stress at a much higher level than the day-to-day concerns.

Stress issues can often build upon one another, creating an exponential effect. Problems that we have faced over the years may seem unrelated when, in actuality, it may be the same basic issue appearing in different forms over and over again. Each time that conflict arises—regardless of the form or shape it takes—it reinforces the source issue with a compounding effect.

An example of this is the woman who has experienced a couple of miscarriages. Miscarriages can clearly instill the fear of losing another baby in a subsequent pregnancy. That *fear of loss* might go much deeper and have roots that began long before the miscarriages. The fear of loss and feeling unsupported may be rooted in feelings of loneliness and abandonment that she experienced as a child as she watched her alcoholic parents disappear emotionally into their drinking. Perhaps, as a teenager, she lost her grandmother, who was the only person in her youth who gave her unconditional love. That generated more feelings of loss and separation. Perhaps there was a relationship in her early twenties where the boyfriend she thought was her true love left her without much explanation. Add to that scenario, trying to have a baby with a husband who can sometimes be "distant." Perhaps he buried himself in his work—at the time of the miscarriages—because he didn't know how to process his own grief or how to support his wife during that difficult time. Not only is there loss and separation from the miscarriages, but those losses are reinforcing a history of loss and separation. The miscarriages, which are tremendously difficult in and of themselves, added to what was already an open wound.

Suddenly, having a family begins to feel scary and uncomfortable at a deep subconscious level. Based on her past experiences, that woman's subconscious mind might believe that if she gets pregnant, she may have to do everything on her own because people in her life have never been there for her with any consistency. For someone in this situation, cutting down on the work hours to lessen her stress may temporarily relieve one component of stress, but it does nothing to relieve the internal accumulation of the deeper, ongoing emotional anxiety.

This example, based on the types of circumstances that I observe with clients, illustrates how the subconscious mind makes connections. In this case, the connections are all related to loss, abandonment, and feeling unsupported. The end result is that those connections generate feelings of anxiety and fear which, in turn, create much of the deep-seated stress that interferes with the process of conception.

We've all heard the cliché: "the issues are in your tissues," which basically means that our bodies are a reflection of our emotions. The significance of that concept is that the issues, and subsequent stress, are a culmination of life experiences and not simply due to our day-to-day activities and workload. The stress from old wounds is always with us until we process and heal it.

Stress—whether it be the day-to-day stuff or the deep subconscious material—is the most significant block to getting pregnant. While there are many familiar ways in which stress can affect our bodies—such as high blood pressure, headaches, insomnia, and ulcers—stress can also be responsible for disrupting hormone production, inadequate blood flow to the uterus, poor follicular quality, and so on. This is because of the way stress affects the functioning of the hypothalamus gland. The focus of this chapter is to examine how emotional issues disrupt the physiology of the body, and, in regards to infertility, how they can turn off the ability to reproduce.

THE HYPOTHALAMUS GLAND
AND HOW IT RESPONDS TO STRESS

The hypothalamus gland (see figure 4.1) is a little gland that sits at the base of the brain. It is considered by many to be the control center of reproductive activity. The hypothalamus doesn't create hormones, but it is the gland that sends out the signals for the body to produce hormones. It is highly sensitive to stress. The signals received by the hypothalamus gland are the starting point for a series of physiological events. Clinical psychologist Dr. Elizabeth Muir explains:

> … the hypothalamus, the neural center at the base of the brain [is] linked to the pituitary gland and controls the flow of hormones in the body. The hypothalamus is sensitive to stress and acts as a bridge between the emotional and physical, turning emotional messages into physical responses that affect hormone levels.[1]

In other words, when our bodies experience stress, the hypothalamus gland takes that emotional signal and generates a physical response that influences the production of hormones.

Niravi Payne, M.S., a psychotherapist who also specializes in fertility work, says that "Emotionally-laden experiences are transmitted biochemically and electrically to the hypothalamus…." The result of that stress, according to Payne, is that it negatively affects "the pituitary gland's output of LH and FSH, affecting ovulation."[2] Luteinizing hormone (LH) and follicle-stimulating hormone (FSH) are two hormones

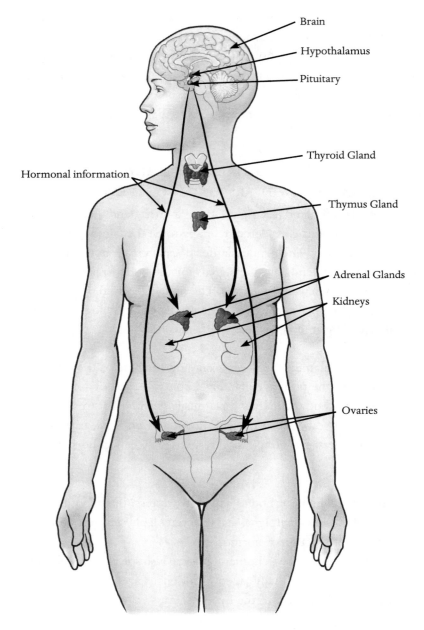

Figure 4.1: The hypothalamus gland and the endocrine system.

directly responsible for a woman's ability to ovulate normally. If these hormones are not in proper balance, ovulation—the release of a mature egg from the ovaries—is interrupted and it is unlikely that conception will take place. Therefore, stress impacts the hypothalamus gland, which, in turn, sends a signal that upsets the balance of hormones released by the pituitary gland. Those unbalanced hormones disrupt ovulation and that creates an infertile situation.

Research from the medical community supports this perspective. According to the Mayo Clinic, when the hypothalamus is stressed, it can create a series of imbalances. This disturbance sets off a chain reaction that can adversely affect the performance of the pituitary gland, hormone production, and ovulation, all of which are key components in creating conception. "Disruption in the part of the brain that regulates ovulation (hypothalamic-pituitary axis) can cause deficiencies in luteinizing hormone (LH) and follicle-stimulating hormone (FSH). Even slight irregularities in the hormone system can affect ovulation."[3]

The significance of the hypothalamus gland and its relationship to fertility isn't just limited to the Western medical belief system. Practitioners of Eastern medicine also focus on the hypothalamic-pituitary-ovarian axis when they work with women who are trying to conceive. Giovanni Maciocia, master teacher of Oriental medicine and author of *Obstetrics and Gynecology in Chinese Medicine*, says that many cases of infertility are "due to a disturbance of the hypothalamic-pituitary-ovarian axis."[4] Maciocia goes on to say that "Alteration of the hypothalamic function may derive from stress, which explains the influence of emotional problems on fertility seen in Chinese medicine."[5]

An example of how stress can affect ovulation and cycles in women is evidenced by the more extreme reactions that occur in women who run marathons. While the marathon runner might physically look toned, and she might say that she feels great, her body is actually under tremendous physical strain. As a reaction to the stress, marathon runners often stop having periods. That response is described by Dr. Aniruddha Malpani and Dr. Anjali Malpani in their book *How to Have a Baby: Overcoming Infertility*:

Excessive stress may even lead to complete suppression of the menstrual cycle, and this is often seen in female marathon runners, who develop "runner's amenorrhea." In less severe cases, it could cause anovulation or irregular menstrual cycles.[6]

The hypothalamus gland, in the case of the marathon runner, behaves as if this woman is running for her life and—in conjunction with other physiological processes—responds by entering a survival, or *fight-or-flight* mode. This response is usually precipitated by feelings of fear, and it causes the blood in our bodies to go mainly to our arms and legs. That way we can fight, if we need to, or run away. Many of us experienced this mode when we were kids, and we ran really fast to get away from whatever was chasing us. Fight-or-flight may help us when we are in danger, but if we look at this in the context of infertility, the blood moves to the extremities and not where it needs to be to promote conception. The woman trying to conceive needs that blood to oxygenate and nourish the internal organs, especially the organs in the reproductive system. The uterus requires a healthy, nurturing flow of blood in the uterine lining to support an implanted embryo.

In addition to the fight-or-flight response, a hypothalamus gland that is registering stress can create another reaction in the body that is very detrimental to the conception process. The hypothalamus can respond to that situation by telling the body to produce cortisol. Cortisol, a stress hormone, is produced by the adrenal glands when we feel anxious or overwhelmed. The combination of the release of cortisol and the fight-or-flight response is extremely unfavorable to conception. It causes the body to go into survival mode, and in survival mode, the physical body is programmed to stay alive, *not to reproduce*.

There are often cases where a woman's hormone levels and cycle are fine—as in many cases of unexplained infertility—but the hypothalamus gland is stressed and telling the body to release cortisol. This, in turn, creates more fear-based fight-or-flight reactions in the body. An example of this, discussed in chapter two, was a female called Rena who participated in the *Psychosomatics* study. As a response to her fear, the muscles around Rena's fallopian tubes would constrict during ovulation, closing the tubes and thereby blocking any chance of pregnancy. In all other ways Rena was a healthy female with the ability to reproduce, but the fear response in her body was causing her infertility.[7] This is an example of how cortisol could be influencing someone who is perfectly healthy and, based on the standard tests for infertility, has no other reason why she can't become pregnant.

It is interesting, and perhaps unfortunate, but the gland that is in control of reproduction is also the gland that is hyper-sensitive to stress. Aniruddha and Anjali Malpani concluded: "Biologically, since the hypothalamus regulates both stress responses as well as the sex hormones, it's easy to see how stress could cause infertility in some women."[8]

It is important to keep in mind that the hypothalamus gland simply responds to stress. It does not differentiate between the enormous physical stress of frequent running, an overwhelming workload or a traumatizing event from the past that is still pushing our buttons. *Even though most fertility clients aren't marathon runners, the level of stress many women are under—from the workplace, from their families, from their past issues and from trying to get pregnant—is not far off from the marathon runner.*

A large segment of our population is operating with elevated cortisol levels and experiencing some degree of fight or flight. Some people might say "fight-or flight doesn't apply to me because it sounds like the feelings of a trapped animal, and I don't feel that way." However, the fight or flight response is, in fact, all those unpleasant feelings, such as being overwhelmed, anxious, and irritable, feelings that are commonly referred to as stress. These feelings get to be so familiar that we learn to live with them and underestimate their impact. In my practice, I find that about four out of five clients have no idea how stressed they are until they enter hypnosis and experience true relaxation.

Any woman who has struggled to conceive will tell you that infertility, with or without medical intervention, is extremely stressful.

THE ON/OFF SWITCH

The hypothalamus gland—acting as the control center in the brain for reproductive activity—can almost be compared to a master switch with an "on" and an "off" position. The information from the hypothalamus affects the autonomic nervous system, the part of the nervous system that controls and regulates numerous functions in the physical body such as the action of heart muscles, digestive functions, hormone production, and normal respiration. The autonomic nervous system has two different modes of operation which are known as the sympathetic and parasympathetic nervous systems. The body will usually engage in one or the other of these two systems. When a woman is calm and feeling relaxed, then the parasympathetic nervous system in her body is turned on. The parasympathetic nervous system, in response to the calm energy, is essentially placing the switch for reproduction into the on position.

Conversely, if a woman is feeling stressed, that engages the sympathetic nervous system. Her body might exhibit some degree of fight-or-flight response and produce cortisol, the stress hormone. Other physiological responses that occur when the sympathetic nervous system is engaged might include an elevated heart rate, higher blood pressure, and constricted blood vessels. (One consequence of constricted blood vessels is insufficient uterine blood flow.) The cumulative result is when the sympathetic nervous system is activated, the switch for reproductive activity essentially moves into the off position. It is yet another way that the status or state of our physiology is directly related to the level of stress or relaxation.

What this means is that women who are under a lot of stress may have the conception switch continually in the off position. They may be trying to get pregnant while the stress they are carrying in their bodies might be rendering much of their infertility procedures and processes ineffective.

A telling sign of this was the study in Israel, discussed in chapter two, where women were split into two groups. Both groups underwent IVF procedures, but one group also received a hypnosis session, to help reduce anxiety around their procedure, at the time of implantation. Twice as many of the women treated with hypnosis got pregnant, compared to those who didn't experience hypnosis.[9] My assumption about this study is that during the single session of hypnosis, some of these women reached a deep-enough level of relaxation that they were temporarily able to switch from the sympathetic response to the parasympathetic response. Engaging the parasympathetic nervous system during that critical time of implantation was key to helping the body reach a state where it could support the conception process. This experiment only included a single hypnosis session performed at the time of implantation. Imagine if the stress reduction work had started a month prior to the IVF procedure and was performed on a regular basis.

HOW STRESS CAN AFFECT AN FSH TEST

A test of a woman's FSH is a blood test used in allopathic medicine to determine how much effort is being expended by a woman's body to produce viable eggs for reproductive purposes. If a woman is not producing quality follicles, her FSH levels increase in an effort to correct the situation. An FSH of 10 or above is generally considered by Western medical doctors to be the point where assisted reproductive technology (ART) is recommended, because it is believed that it is unlikely a woman can conceive naturally once her FSH reaches that threshold.

To better understand the relationship between FSH and follicular quality, a comparison can be made to the performance of the thyroid gland and TSH, the thyroid-stimulating hormone. When a thyroid gland is underperforming, the TSH increases because the function of the thyroid stimulating hormone is to stimulate the thyroid to work harder. Thus, a blood test that shows a high TSH level indicates that the thyroid is not functioning at optimum levels and, as a result, the hormones are trying to push the thyroid to boost its performance. The relationship between FSH and follicular quality is very similar: high FSH means that the body is generating a higher level of the hormone responsible for the production of viable eggs in order to compensate for a reproductive system that is underperforming.

However, as described above, *FSH is strongly impacted by stress, so a woman who is experiencing high stress levels may not get an accurate read on her fertility situation based on an FSH test.* A woman in a highly stressful situation—whether that is related to work, family, issues from her past, or even the incredible pressure of undergoing tests to see if she will be able to have children—is very likely to have elevated FSH levels due to the increased anxiety she is experiencing. In other words, a woman who might normally have an FSH that falls within the acceptable range may find that her FSH becomes elevated simply because of her anxiety.

This is why many practitioners of alternative modalities *strongly dispute* using FSH as a conclusive marker when treating infertility. The primary reason for this is a simple fact: *before an accurate FSH diagnosis can be ascertained, the stress levels must be brought into an acceptable range.* It is extremely rare that a woman is provided with this information before submitting to the blood test.

The other reason why FSH should not be considered *the* determining factor in how to address the infertility picture is because of the success that practitioners of Eastern medicine have had in working with FSH issues. With acupuncture and herbs, the low performance of the reproductive system that is creating the elevated FSH level can be treated and brought into balance. For example, if the ovaries are not generating viable follicles, the approach of Eastern medicine is to use the natural energy within the body to boost the performance of the ovaries, which, in turn, can positively affect the quality of the follicles. Acupuncture can also be helpful in reducing stress. It is quite common to see a woman's FSH level go down after working with an Eastern medicine practitioner.

Another valuable tool in this process is the utilization of mind-body healing (discussed in chapter 9) where a woman employs meditation and mind-body healing techniques to increase the functioning of the reproductive system so that it operates at a higher level. Mind-body healing and meditation are both beneficial methods of reducing stress.

Before a woman undergoes an FSH test, I recommend the following:

1. Lower her stress to a manageable level by working with meditation and processing the interfering subconscious issues.

2. Work with acupuncture and herbs to ensure that her reproductive system is energetically balanced.

3. Utilize mind-body techniques to have her body and reproductive system working at optimum levels.

Only then can her true FSH level be ascertained. Without doing that work, it is likely that the result might be an elevated FSH level, and that high FSH score may prompt a decision to employ assisted reproductive techniques when a natural conception may be a very realistic alternative.

STRESS IN OUR SOCIETY

As I mentioned earlier, we feel stress from our jobs, our bills, our past embedded issues, our families, and so on, but we also live in a society where fear—which generates enormous stress—is constantly used for purposes of control and manipulation. If we sit down and watch the news—or the teasers between programs to get viewers interested in watching the news—how many of those stories are designed to provoke interest by tapping into our fears? When the stock market undergoes a big drop, what is driving the panicked sell-off? When we make decisions about what type and how much insurance we buy, how does that salesperson get us to spend a few more dollars? When politicians try to get votes by telling us that their opponent can't protect us from the "evils of the world," how are they trying to use manipulation to get your vote? Even the corporate world has us believing that they are taking care of us, with wages and benefits, and if we quit our jobs, how in the world could we survive on our own?

We are being constantly bombarded by messages of fear; therefore, it is important to look at how we are responding to these messages. Probably the best way to deal with the stress that comes from fearful stimuli is to keep things in perspective and not get drawn in or become engaged by giving into those fears. We can start by reducing our exposure to the news media. While we may need enough information to make informed decisions when we vote in elections, an ongoing barrage of stories about murders, assaults, kidnappings, etc. takes away from our ability to stay in a relaxed, happy state of mind. Be selective about violent movies and television. As we become more conscious of this, we can develop a strategy where we become more discriminating about what external stress-provoking stimuli we choose to allow into our lives.

Try to embrace the belief that you are always loved and protected. Remember the law of attraction: *what you think about and believe is what you attract to yourself.* If you believe that you are safe and cared for, then that is the energy that is always around you as you move through life. This mindset is far more conducive to creating a low stress environment where conception can more easily be attainable.

HOW TO DEAL WITH STRESS

There are many techniques—in addition to not participating in fear-based thinking—for stress reduction. Some of those include breathing exercises, visualization, meditation, yoga (not hot or extreme yoga), hypnosis, biofeedback, massage, acupuncture, and gentle exercise. It is important to spend a part of every day working with some form of relaxation technique because it is easy for stressful responses to be running our biology without our full awareness.

WORKING WITH THE MEDITATIONS
IN THIS BOOK

I provide several meditations in this book. Many of them are designed to simply help you take stock of or observe your present state or condition. The meditation for this chapter is a way for you to go inside and evaluate your level of calmness based on what you observe from your hypothalamus gland. If you discover that there is much internal stress, then that is an indication that a relaxation technique, such as those listed above, would be beneficial for you.

Be creative and imaginative. Sometimes, when we first start to meditate, the images we create or imagine last for only a second or two, or they may seem kind of vague. That is okay. Just tune in to what you imagined for that brief moment and be aware of any feelings or information that might have accompanied that image.

It is best to do these meditations with a partner so that you can focus and not have to keep interrupting the process by looking at the book.*

---

* If you don't have a partner to read the meditations to you, you can purchase an audio recording that contains all of the meditations from this book at www.themindbodyconnection.com.

After you get comfortable and relaxed, ask your partner to read the meditation to you. Begin each meditation by closing your eyes and taking a few deep breaths. Naturally, meditation should never be done while driving or participating in activities that require our full attention. It is best to turn off all phones and electronic devices so that there won't be any interruptions.

HYPOTHALAMUS MEDITATION

Close your eyes and take a few deep breaths to help you relax.

Imagine that you are stepping into a small room. There is a red button on the wall with the letter *S* on it. When you press that button, you will become very small (just like *Alice in Wonderland*). Press the button when you are ready and imagine becoming very small, maybe one inch tall. After you become tiny, look around and you will notice a small door or opening, about the same size as a mouse hole. In a moment when you walk through that opening, you will find yourself standing at the base of your brain with your hypothalamus gland right in front of you. Observe the hypothalamus as being about the size of a basketball. When you are ready, imagine yourself walking through the door and stepping right up to your hypothalamus gland.

Observe your hypothalamus. Does it look relaxed? Is the color of the hypothalamus bright or dull? For those of you who like to touch, you might get a better sense of whether your hypothalamus is relaxed or stressed by putting your hands right on it and feeling its texture and energy. Is it tense or calm? Does it look bright and full of vigor? Is it tired? Does it need to be rejuvenated? Take your time and be open to whatever information presents itself. (Pause for a few minutes to make observations.)

After making your inspection, go back through the little hole into the small room. You will see a button with an *L*, for large, on it. Press that button and imagine your body getting larger until it becomes normal-sized again. Take a few deep breaths, then gently open your eyes. You might want to write down your observations.

In Their Own Words

Emily's story shows how stress can affect reproductive functions. Much of her stress was connected to a miscarriage, but there was also a great deal of fear creating deep-seated anxiety. By processing and releasing the blocking issues, Emily was able to significantly reduce her stress and switch her body from the sympathetic stress mode to the parasympathetic relaxed mode.

Emily's Story
Healing from the Trauma of Miscarriage

My husband and I had "unexplained infertility" and we had been trying to conceive for over ten years. We began the conception process by going off the pill in June of 1998. After two years of not being able to conceive, we proceeded to do intrauterine inseminations (IUI) for about six cycles. No pregnancies resulted from those procedures. After a period of time, we decided to proceed with an IVF. In March of 2004, we did a fresh IVF cycle, implanting four eggs with one leftover, and again, no pregnancy resulted. I did not do anything additional with this first IVF cycle except for the standard IVF process: no mind-body treatments and no acupuncture. Unfortunately, with only one egg in frozen storage it is not typically recommended to attempt a frozen cycle.

We were, of course, devastated at our inability to conceive after the first IVF cycle. It took us over a year to get the nerve up to repeat another fresh cycle. In the meantime, I began receiving acupuncture regularly in the hope that I could conceive naturally. In August of 2005, we proceeded with our second fresh IVF cycle. Again, we had four eggs implanted and had one leftover embryo which was frozen for possible future use. At this IVF cycle, we did conceive a son, whom we lost at twenty-one weeks for no apparent reason. I had to have an emergency C-section due to extreme blood loss, to save my life, but it resulted in the death of our son, as his lungs were not developed. After the C-section I was not allowed medically to get pregnant for six to twelve months.

In November of 2006, I was still getting regular acupuncture treatments. It was at that time I started working with hypnotherapy to address my fears and concerns about losing our son, and the concerns about getting pregnant again and the toll that would take on my psyche.

The hypnosis helped me to visualize my future with a child, to address my fears in a visual/emotional way, to create a positive outlook, and really foresee myself becoming pregnant. It gave me the ability to really see myself going through the pregnancy, giving birth, and also seeing my child in the future.

The biggest issue for me was the fear of having another miscarriage, but we had to work through several other issues. There was the fear of failure, the fear of loss, the fear of the changes in my body during and after pregnancy, the fear of my ability to go through nine to ten months on pins and needles as we waited to see about viability, and even fear of the birth process itself. These were all issues that needed to be processed so I could be at peace before starting another procedure.

Hypnotherapy changed my life. I went from fearful to excited. It was an incredible transformation: I went from cynic to the most positive person possible. I felt like it was Christmas on my transfer day. My husband was astounded by the change in my attitude.

Finally, in late November of 2006, after receiving the all clear from my doctor, we implanted the two frozen embryos left over from our two previous IVF cycles. In July of 2007, as a result of the frozen transfer, I gave birth to a beautiful baby girl. It was the hypnosis, in conjunction with acupuncture, that I believe cinched my pregnancy and gave me the tools to use when I became fearful. I was able to meditate on specific issues, and as those issues changed or new ones arose, I saw my hypnotherapist and we would change the meditation accordingly.

Hypnotherapy was the key to managing my expectations and helping me progress through my pregnancy at various points when issues such as resentfulness due to exhaustion and nausea (yet still thrilled about the pregnancy!) and, naturally, a fear of loss at the twenty-one-week mark because of memories from the past. It was extremely helpful, and I would recommend it highly for anyone in my situation because the mind can be difficult to control when it is under the kind of stress that comes not only with fertility procedures but also after the loss of a pregnancy.

WORKS CITED

1. Suzy Greaves, "Can Hypnosis Help to Make You Pregnant." *The Times Newspapers* (TimesOnLine.com) Mar. 5, 2002.
2. Ibid.
3. Mayo Foundation for Medical Education and Research (MFMER). "Diseases and Conditions: Infertility" From *MayoClinic.com*. June 15, 2006.
4. Giovanni Maciocia, *Obstetrics and Gynecology in Chinese Medicine* (New York, New York: Churchill Livingstone, 1998), 735.
5. Ibid. 735–6.
6. Dr. Aniruddha Malpani, and Dr. Anjali Malpani, "How to Have a Baby: Overcoming Infertility." http://www.fertilitycommunity.com/fertility/32-stress-and-infertility.html Chapter 32, 1.
7. Howard R. Lewis, and Martha E. Lewis, *Psychosomatics* (New York, New York: Pinnacle Books, 1972), 210–211.
8. Malpani, "How to Have a Baby," Chapter 32, 1.
9. David Brinn, "Israeli study proves hypnosis can double IVF success rate." Our Jerusalem, http://www.ourjerusalem.com/news/story/news20040824.html, Aug. 22, 2004.

CHAPTER FIVE

ISSUES AND EMOTIONS THAT
BLOCK CONCEPTION

It is easy to see how stress in our workplace or unhealthy family dynamics can cause us to feel overwhelmed, tired, irritable, and anxious, and we understand how this can affect our fertility, but several thousand years ago, the Chinese observed that women who had difficulty conceiving often had an underlying emotional issue that was preventing conception. This concept, which had been ignored for centuries, is now regarded as a significant piece of the infertility picture. We no longer look at infertility as simply a biological process. Instead it is a much more complicated culmination of the mind and body working together to create life. Dr. Christiane Northrup, in her book *Women's Bodies, Women's Wisdom,* talked about the importance of a healthy mind as being a significant factor in the conception process. Northrup wrote: "Regardless of what you've been told about your fertility, you need to know that your ability to conceive is profoundly influenced by the complex interaction among psychosocial, psychological, and emotional factors, and that you can consciously work with this to enhance your ability to have a baby."[1] Our thoughts, feelings, and beliefs have a direct impact on the biology within our bodies. For many woman, the process of healing the emotional issues that are blocking pregnancy is a key component in unlocking fertility and opening the door to conception.

The body and the mind work as a synchronistic team. When both are in balance, the process of conception can begin. Unfortunately, many people place all of the emphasis in their efforts to conceive strictly on the physical elements, and underestimate the power of the mind.

Studies documented in chapter two of this book indicate that psychological and emotional blocks appear to be the root of many infertility situations. Those studies showed—through the success rates of patients who worked directly with the psychological elements—that as the negative emotions and issues were processed, conception rates increased dramatically.

Dr. Elizabeth Muir, a clinical psychologist based in London who specializes in treating infertility, says, "I believe that while a woman might consciously want a baby, her subconscious may be stopping her from getting pregnant. Most women I see have psychosomatic infertility related to conflicts or unresolved issues about having a baby."[2] It is those conflicts or unresolved issues that send a message to the body—and the cells—that interferes with the process. (See chapter eight for more information about cellular messages.)

When the mind and emotions are in a state of turbulence or unrest, the mind-body connection becomes out of sync, resulting in negative physiological responses. Dr. Andrew Weil addresses this situation in his book called *Spontaneous Healing*: "... the mind can depress the immune system and can unbalance the autonomic nervous system, leading to disturbances in digestion, circulation, and all other internal functions. You must know how to use the mind in the service of healing."[3] Weil is saying that the mind can work for us or against us. When one feels free of the issues that are weighing them down, then their mind can become a strong ally in getting pregnant. Conversely, a mind that is bogged down by fears, stressful thoughts, and negative emotions is too overwhelmed to communicate positive messages to the body.

How can emotional issues create feelings of distress and, in turn, cause infertility? It is deep within the subconscious mind where all of the emotional issues and blocks related to infertility are stored. As discussed in chapter three, the subconscious mind holds our habits, beliefs, behavioral patterns, anxieties, and fears that we have been accumulating since birth. Then, as adults, when we experience emotions like anxiety, sadness, fear, or anger, we are responding to the cumulative effect of the information and programming that has collected throughout our entire lifetime.

Negative feelings and emotions within the subconscious can intensify and become all-consuming to the woman experiencing infertility. An experience from years past, such as a feeling of failure, can become so intense that it can control our present belief system without us even knowing it. These old emotions feed our current fears: "Why is this happening to me: is it something I did in my past?" "I feel like I'm letting everyone in the family down." "What if I fail again in this cycle?" "Maybe I don't deserve a child." "I'm so afraid of having another miscarriage." "What if I never have a child?" These fears and insecurities are often connected to old unhealed emotions. If those unhealed emotional issues are disregarded, it can disrupt the mind-body connection and lead to feelings of disharmony and stress, both of which are major blocks to conception.

The positive news about these blocks is that they can be healed or processed. That means addressing issues that some of us wish would just go away. The reality is that our emotional stuff won't just go away. We need to clean out the residue by doing the emotional work. The reward for that work is life-changing: feelings of confidence, joy, and emotional well-being, and the creation of a mindset that is at peace and ready to have a baby.

THE COMMON BLOCKS TO CONCEPTION

What are the most common mental and emotional blocks to conception? Based on years of work with infertility clients, I've compiled a list of the most common issues and patterns I've observed with women struggling to get pregnant (see page 73).

The fact that issues can become hidden or buried in the subconscious mind makes the process of identifying those issues much more complicated. In a session, I can ask someone face-to-face how they feel about something and then check out that same situation in hypnosis— where the answer is coming directly from the subconscious—and often get two very different responses. That is because one of those responses is being filtered by the conscious mind, and the other is unfiltered and honest. For example, I might ask a woman if she thinks that there are any family issues that might be creating interference with her ability to conceive. She might say that she has always been at odds with her mother, but they have finally reached a point where they now can be civil toward each other. Then, in hypnosis, much more information may be revealed. It is quite common for an emotional response to occur in a situation like that because the feelings related to her mother may have been held inside for years and never expressed. In the session, it might be revealed that her mother always made her feel not good enough or not worthy. That woman, during the session, might remember a time she had consciously forgotten where her mother, in a moment of anger, told her, "you just can't do anything right, can you." Or perhaps her mother, in an effort to exercise control and make sure her daughter will always consider her mother's feelings before her own, may have been more direct with her words by saying something like "you're too selfish to have kids." All of this information—stored in the subconscious mind—creates a tape that continually plays deep within our being and programs how we feel and what we believe about ourselves. That tape, for this woman, will make her question, at a very deep level, if she really *can* be a good mother and if she truly *is* worthy or deserving to have kids. It isn't uncommon for the woman to have completely forgotten both the words and the encounter with her mother until it emerges from her subconscious memory during hypnosis. As a client recalls information like this, they typically respond by saying, "I hadn't thought about that day in years, but now as it comes back, I remember how devastated I was when she said that." Sometimes, all a woman will consciously *know* about that programming is that there is something inside of her that wants to prove her mother wrong, adding additional pressure to get pregnant. This woman's logical mind might say "of course I can be a good mother," but the subconscious programming is far more powerful than what the critical mind wants to believe.

The key point is that the information that needs to be processed and reprogrammed is within the subconscious—not the conscious—mind. In other words, *we can't just consciously think or remember or identify what issues are interfering with conception. That information can only be accessed from the subconscious mind.* Most women will look at the list of blocks in this chapter and pick out two or three items that they know apply to them. Later, when they work with the subconscious mind, there are often a couple of different issues that are revealed. We can never predict if it will be the hidden issues that will create major disruptions, or the ones we know but underestimate—as in the example above—that are interfering with the ability to conceive.

Some clients want to do this work but are afraid that some dark, repressed experience, such as sexual abuse, will be revealed. That is almost never the case. It is true that sometimes people will block out memories of the actual experiences of sexual abuse, but those clients almost always come in and say that they are pretty sure that "something occurred when they were young." In other words, people usually have a feeling that something abusive may have happened in their past. If this is the case, an issue of that magnitude will need to be addressed. However, if there are no indications or suspicions coming from the conscious mind, *it is extremely rare for a traumatic memory to come out of nowhere* while working with the subconscious mind. The more common scenario is what I described above where a woman may have greatly underestimated the power of the experience, such as the importance that her mother's words might have had on her ability to conceive. She might have had an awareness or some level of discomfort about the relationship, but she didn't know to what extent it was affecting her. *By opening up to the subconscious programming, we get a very accurate picture of the emotional charge of the various issues that may be residing there, and it is those powerful feelings that become blocks to fertility.*

We never know how powerful an emotional block really is until we work directly with the subconscious mind, because no two people respond the same way to the same concern. An issue for one woman can be the cause of a great deal of discomfort, while that same issue may not even elicit a response from another woman. An example of that might be body-image concerns. Sometimes, in hypnosis, I'll have a woman stand in front of a mirror and imagine her body at eight months of pregnancy. Some women who do this will instantly become very uncomfortable. A woman who has always prided herself in keeping in perfect shape might suddenly see her body changing in ways that she feels might make her unattractive and imperfect. Women with this concern will sometimes twist and turn anxiously in their chair and want nothing to do with that body they just imagined. Had I asked about body image before the session, or looked at the questionnaire women fill out before they see me, that might not have been considered as a possible issue.

It is very difficult to know the true level of the emotional response until we access the information at the source. Subconscious feelings and beliefs can go undetected and subsequently become unidentified blocks to fertility. That woman with the body image concerns may never realize the degree to which that fear is getting in the way of what she wants most in life. As long as it is undetected, the block remains in place. Her mind and body are at odds with each other. Deep down, conception and pregnancy might elicit a very uncomfortable feeling, a feeling that may be causing physiological responses—such as the stress responses described in chapter four—that make it impossible for her to get pregnant. Even if that woman resorts to a medical procedure such as an IVF, she may still have trouble getting pregnant or maintaining the pregnancy because the body image block is still in place.

MIND-BODY BLOCKS

In addition to body image, what other fears or issues or blocks might be powerful enough to keep a woman from conceiving? There may be subconscious issues around pregnancy, labor, childbirth, hospitals, medical treatments, motherhood, loss of independence, questions about their husband's ability to be a good father, unresolved dysfunctional patterns from a woman's own childhood, worries about balancing a family and a career, or simply the fear of failure to conceive under the financial and psychological pressure that comes with medical reproductive procedures.

It is important to note, we do not have to reprogram every negative emotional experience we have ever had. We all have dozens, maybe hundreds of these. While it may be true that our personal growth in this lifetime is dependent on how conscious we decide to become, it is *not imperative to heal everything* before conception can occur. It is necessary, however, to heal those major obstacles standing in the way of pregnancy. The innate wisdom of the subconscious mind knows what these issues are and will bring those forward. We have the rest of our days to investigate the things that may be holding us back in other areas of our lives.

Issues that are blocks to conception:

- Sexual abuse

- Rape

- Miscarriages

- Abortions

- Dysfunctional family relationships (birth family)

- Pressure of perfectionism

- Concern about body image/physical changes to her body

- Concern about trying to balance a career and family

- Self-doubt: Will she be a good mother?

- Self-doubt: Is she ready to be a mother?

- Fear of failure

- Fear of labor and childbirth

- Fear of hospitals

- Fear of medical treatments

- Fear of loss of independence and individuality

- Concern about her husband being a good father

- Concern about the new baby being a threat to the marital relationship

While this list is certainly not all-inclusive, it does include some of the most common and most debilitating blocks in terms of how they can derail one's ability to get pregnant. The top six are the ones that present the most formidable obstacles. I find it extremely rare that someone is able to conceive if they are presenting one of the top six issues and don't do any processing or healing around that concern. It is possible, but in my observation, it isn't likely.

A BRIEF DISCUSSION OF THE ISSUES

I won't go into a detailed discussion of the issues of sexual abuse and rape because they are self-explanatory. Since they hold such a strong emotional charge, it goes without saying that those two concerns need to be addressed. The focus of this book is not about the treatment of sexual abuse, but the impact of that experience will usually create a great deal of fear and stress, both of which become substantial blocks to fertility. Healing the emotions from these types of situations can shift the body out of the stress mode and into a place of fertile receptivity.

Some of the other top issues—miscarriages, abortions, and dysfunctional family relationships—are discussed in the remainder of this chapter. Perfectionism is important enough that an entire chapter of this book is devoted to that subject alone. Most of the remaining items on the list have their roots in one basic emotion: fear. Fear, discussed in depth in the next chapter, is the feeling that most often triggers the stress response.

Miscarriages

Everyone loves to talk about their success stories—how exciting it is having babies—but few talk openly about miscarriages, a very common occurrence that many women have endured before having a successful pregnancy. Statistics vary widely in regard to the likelihood of a pregnancy ending in miscarriage: I have seen numbers that range from 20 to 60 percent for women in the 35–45-year-old age group. It appears that the higher number may be closer to the truth. Probably two-thirds of the women I see in my office have had at least one—often two—miscarriages.

The number of pregnancies that don't go full-term is very high, but for most women it is too painful to revisit and too difficult to talk about, so it makes sense that few women wish to share information about their pregnancies that ended prematurely. As a result, many women who have a miscarriage feel that they may be in the minority and something is wrong with them. In truth, it probably means quite the opposite: they are very normal.

It is important to understand that not only are miscarriages fairly common, but it is nature's way of stepping in when something is wrong. When our biology perceives an insurmountable deficiency, it responds by bringing an end to the pregnancy.

It is common for a woman who has had a miscarriage to be overwhelmed by negative feelings and emotions. Many women respond with feelings of not being good enough or assuming something must be wrong with them. Another reaction that sometimes occurs is guilt as a woman racks her brain to try to figure out what she did wrong, either during her pregnancy or in the past. Sometimes that woman will even assume that she is paying for past sins. Those women who are struggling with high expectations or perfectionism might experience feelings of failure, and often put even more pressure on themselves—thereby creating an even larger barrier to fertility—as they become more determined to *make sure* there is success next time. (See chapter seven for more information on perfectionism.)

Whether the experience brings up guilt, inadequacy, or the fear of failure, the anxiety around having another miscarriage often becomes immense. Unless the miscarriage occurs so early that the woman wasn't even sure she was pregnant, most women start establishing a connection to the baby growing inside them early on, and there is an overwhelming sense of grief when that connection is lost. Therefore it is important to take time for grieving and processing. This usually necessitates working with a practitioner because having this type of loss is an emotionally charged event. When there are unhealed emotions—whether it be inadequacy, guilt, or fear—the resulting stress can shut down the body's ability to conceive. (See chapter four about stress and infertility.)

Due to the emotional aspects of miscarriages and abortions, these two issues present two of the biggest blocks to fertility. The good news is that once they are processed, these two issues usually have a fast turnaround time. In other words, once that work is done, it is common for women to conceive fairly soon.

Abortions

While miscarriages create powerful emotional blocks in women trying to conceive, they don't seem to come close to matching the issue of abortion when it comes to interfering with the conception process. Abortions rank as one of the biggest blocks to fertility. The guilt from having an abortion is immense. It can come from society, the beliefs and attitudes of our birth families, the religious background under which we were raised, or current religious beliefs and morals. All of those factors can create self-imposed guilt that gets buried in the subconscious mind and creates a barrier between the woman and a potential new baby.

Many women, after having an abortion, believe and expect that they will be—and should be—punished by God or whatever figure of divine authority was part of their belief system when they were growing up. Even if they have long since abandoned that belief system, the original religious upbringing seems to have the most power over our thoughts. This is because in our youth our subconscious mind absorbed lots of information without the filtering system that we have developed as adults. Much of the information we learn as kids becomes our law and essentially governs our thoughts and feelings throughout our lives. If that law is such that a woman has never been able to completely forgive herself, then the sense of guilt and self-punishment create an insurmountable wall in the psyche that won't allow the physical body to become pregnant.

I often see women who have spent years—sometimes decades—trying to use penance or prayer to eliminate the emotional charge that comes with an abortion. In the great majority of those cases, it appears that the emotional charge is still there and in full force. Again, the best recourse is to work with a practitioner who can help in this area. Some women decide to never tell anyone about the termination, but trying to heal this without assistance appears to be a nearly impossible task. Some women believe, in their *conscious* minds, that they have moved past this experience, yet in session, this issue will not only come up right away, but it will elicit a very strong emotional response.

The purpose of this discussion is not to take any political, religious, or moral stand on abortion, it is simply to look at various blocks to pregnancy and why it is important to process those blocks. Abortion is a reality, and it might be the most formidable obstacle to achieving pregnancy. Slightly under half of the women I see for infertility have had an abortion, and I have seen very, very few who have had successful pregnancies without doing any work around self-forgiveness to heal that old emotional material.

Dysfunctional Family Relationships

Many women express a deep-seated concern that they may repeat some of their familial dysfunctions. These can include the obvious forms of physical or emotional abuse as well as more subtle family dynamics. Issues such as low self-esteem, feelings of inadequacy, favoritism, patterns of substance abuse, and codependency often create emotional scars in the subconscious mind that may require inner resolution and healing before conception can take place.

A negative belief system, a poor self-concept or even challenging family experiences can become deeply ingrained when we are children and then become a part of our psychological make-up as we become adults. Unfortunately, we don't shed all of the family issues when we move out of the house or away from the birth family. In fact, unless these dysfunctions are identified and processed, it is likely for us to re-experience those same issues, in a little different form, in our adult lives. For example, an abusive and domineering father might be replaced by an abusive and domineering boss or husband. The daughter of a controlling and manipulative mother might express those same qualities after many years of being subjected to that behavior. The old saying about how we marry—or become—our parents is true; however, this has nothing to do with hair color, body type, or other physical traits. Instead, we are expressing and perpetuating many of the dysfunctions that existed in the birth family by our own self-expression or through the partners we choose. Usually, we are unaware of how we are acting that out.

I believe that there are lessons we are supposed to learn during our lifetime. We learn these through many of the relationships we attract and then by addressing and resolving the issues that surface in our relationships. Until they are resolved and we have learned what we are supposed to learn, our issues will continually resurface and create challenges. An example of this, which I often see in infertility work, is the woman who has had a couple of boyfriends, followed by a husband, where she thinks she can fix whatever issues those partners have going on in their lives. She may see a lot of promise in these individuals and believe that she can be the one to help resolve the shortcomings or weaknesses. This is often born out of being the caretaker, the peacemaker, or the person who was trying to fix one of her parents or siblings. Quite often, at a deep level, the partners who have come into her life may not want to be fixed. In her determination to be successful, she will expend a great deal of her emotional energy and it is unlikely that she will ever see those corrections come to fruition.

How can a situation like this affect fertility? First of all, if that woman's husband has an issue that is fairly significant—such as being controlling and manipulative—the struggle to conceive may be impeded by concerns about whether or not her husband will be a good father. If these traits were present in her birth family, she may have deep-seated memories and fears that she and her husband might mirror the relationship that was played out by her parents. She might remember wanting attention or acknowledgement from her father and then feeling empty and rejected when he was correcting and criticizing everything she did. *All of this information becomes a part of the infertility mindset: not just the current situation, but also the memories that originated in childhood.* If fertility was strictly a biological process, these things wouldn't matter, but for millions of women around the world struggling with unexplained infertility, the mental and emotional factors from childhood and birth families *are* a significant part of the fertility picture.

Our experience of family behavior is what we gained firsthand in our childhood. Our subconscious minds have recorded what was modeled for us, and this shapes a lot of our attitudes around having children. Since these old beliefs and patterns become part of the emotional equation when it comes time to start a family, reshaping and reframing some of the old familial programming helps us remove resistance and conquer fear of replicating the past.

Body Image

While the six issues we've just considered are the ones that create the biggest blocks, everyone is different. Sometimes an issue like body image can be a major obstacle. It often begins at an early age, in a woman who participated in dance, gymnastics, cheerleading, athletics or a similar activity where body image was emphasized. What happens here is that a rigid idea of the only acceptable weight, body shape, and fat percentage becomes firmly established. That may have served her in her youth, but now it does not allow for the softness and receptivity in her mature female body that is needed for conception. Reshaping these beliefs is often necessary before she can allow the image of her pregnant body to become a comfortable part of her mindset. As long as her conscious and subconscious minds are in disagreement about this issue it is difficult for her physical body to accept a pregnancy. Body image is often problematic for women who are perfectionists (see chapter seven for more information about perfectionism).

Balancing a Family and a Career

For many women, the dilemma of how to balance a family and career can create mixed signals. Inside, she longs to have a baby, but the part of her that has worked so hard to build a career is not willing to let go. In many of those cases, a compromise can be reached, but if she continues to work fifty to sixty hours a week, accompanied by a vague promise of slowing down *"when* I get pregnant," it indicates that the issue hasn't been resolved. Nothing has changed for her. She is still sending the same signal to her body: her priorities are clearly drawn, and work will continue to draw the majority of her attention and energy.

Self-doubt, Fears, and Concerns

Many of the remaining doubts and concerns on the conception blocks list are connected to various fears, a topic that will be discussed in more detail in the next chapter. In regard to self-doubt, a woman might question whether or not she can be a good mother. The idea of taking care of a newborn can feel a little bit scary. This doubt is often something that grows out of feelings of inadequacy, a feeling which is fairly common in our society. Another set of circumstances that can generate this doubt is when a woman comes from a dysfunctional family situation and is concerned that the old uncomfortable dynamics might arise again, whether it be in the same form as what she experienced or perhaps with a slightly different twist.

A woman will sometimes question if she is ready to be a mother. Sometimes she will wonder if she has accomplished the things she set out to do before settling down to have a family, or she may question if she has the life experience to handle the situations that come with being a parent. Again, these thoughts usually grow out of old buried feelings of inadequacy.

The fear of failure I refer to on the list is not so much about the woman being a terrible mother—which occasionally can be a concern—it is more about failing to ever have children. Some women are afraid that if they aren't able to have children, the people in their life—their parents, in-laws, husband, and friends—will always be disappointed with them. For some, growing up in a family unit teaches us to value procreation and we may fear growing old alone or being uncared for in our elder years. The woman with this mindset may put a great deal of pressure on herself to try to conceive, and that additional pressure only impacts the situation in a negative way.

Some women are afraid of going through labor and childbirth. Given the way that birthing is portrayed in movies and television, as a source of incredible pain, this is no surprise. Additionally, some women have witnessed a birth that may or may not have gone well. These fears need to be unearthed and reframed in a positive way. It is important to note that women can now take classes that teach them how to prepare for birthing through the use of relaxation tools, breathing techniques, and forms of meditation or self-hypnosis. Woman who have prepared themselves for birth by taking classes and practicing these techniques usually find that having a baby can be a wonderful, empowering experience.

The fear of hospitals usually stems from old memories and experiences. Most of us have a memory of pain associated with the hospital. The fear of abandonment can also be associated with hospitals: when a young child is a patient in the hospital and the parents aren't there with them, the child often starts to wonder if the family has left them there. Naturally, the parents can't be with that child every minute, but a young child may not understand that. The other association some people have with hospitals can be that people die in hospitals. Whether it is fear of abandonment, or pain or dying, just imagining that environment can create anxiety in a lot of people.

The fear of medical treatments overlaps with many of the fears that are associated with hospitals. Most people are concerned with the discomfort while others worry that some error or mistake could cause a permanent injury or an early demise. This is a situation where meditation or self-hypnosis can be extremely valuable as a way to counteract those fears.

Some women like to be free to do what they want and go where they want without being tied down by obligations. The independence and freedom that most of us value can change overnight when a baby comes into the picture. Another aspect to this is that one's individual identity often becomes overshadowed by having a baby, because the newborn becomes the new center of attention. Many women are okay with the shift of focus that is now centered around the baby, but sometimes that loss of freedom and identity can be problematic.

Husband and Relationship Concerns

Husband issues can sometimes be a source of difficulty. The most common situation is when the husband is not really sure he wants children. Occasionally women aren't confident that the husband will be good with children or if their spouse will actively participate in the raising of the kids. A few sessions of couples' counseling can usually help bring peace of mind in these areas. Many times it is a matter of opening up communication and working on solutions that are acceptable to everyone. For example, the husband who is worried that his wife will neglect him and give all the attention to the baby might simply be reacting to the memories of neglect from his own childhood. He may need to air his fears and be reassured that this will not be the case. Perhaps the couple can take steps to make sure this doesn't become a problem by doing things such as agreeing to have at least one date night a month where the focus is on keeping their relationship strong.

HOW TO IDENTIFY AND PROCESS
THE BLOCKS

The diagnosis of unexplained infertility implies that the body is healthy and could conceive if thoughts, beliefs, and emotions weren't interfering with the process, so it would follow that addressing these factors is the key to being successful in this work. Most clients I see might have one or two minor physical concerns, but it is usually the emotional baggage that is getting in the way.

How do we identify the hidden issues and do the healing work? As stated in chapter two, in order to identify the subconscious material, hypnosis is probably the most efficient process because it is designed to specifically do this type of work and access the subconscious mind, where our entire emotional history lies. People who have been practicing meditation for many years may be able to unearth some of the blocks, but the meditator should be working with someone in order to process what arises, so it does not expose a wound without the possibility of closure. It is incredibly difficult—and often a type of denial—when we attempt to heal ourselves. *Intense* psychotherapy that elicits deep emotional responses, followed by processing and healing, may also address the blocks. It is extremely unlikely that deep-seated subconscious information will come to light in normal conversations such as ordinary talk therapy, prayer, or support groups. This is because normal discussions are a process of the *conscious* mind, *not the subconscious* mind.

There are always new emotional healing techniques that promise the client that they can do their processing without ever having to directly address the issues. For true healing to take place, one *does* have to work directly with the issues and the foundation of those issues. Avoiding the root or source is essentially a form of denial. Any process where the true source is only vaguely addressed or bypassed entirely is highly unlikely to create any deep emotional healing or lasting success. While positive affirmations may make us feel better in the short term, they don't have the capacity to change the programming of the subconscious.

For those who feel uneasy when thinking about engaging in this kind of work, know that a practitioner who is well trained can help a client work directly with their issues *without* making the client relive the old events. For example, someone who experienced sexual abuse *does not* have to relive or re-experience those events, but they do need to do some healing work around what transpired.

Dr. Deepak Chopra, who has brought much awareness to the importance of the mind-body connection, wrote: "To change the printout of the body, you must learn to rewrite the software of the mind ..."[4] and that "anything in your body can be changed with the flick of an intention."[5] In other words, our minds control what happens in our physical bodies and if we can heal the software—or programming of the subconscious—then we can change what happens within our bodies.

In *Women's Bodies, Women's Wisdom*, Dr. Christiane Northrup describes mind-body work in relation to creating fertility: "The mind-body approach to fertility is based on the premise that knowledge is power and that a change in perception based on new information is powerful enough to effect subtle changes in your endocrine, immune, and nervous systems."[6] We can change our perception by doing the emotional work and healing the old wounds, and that new perception not only opens the door to conception, but it can permanently change our lives in a very positive way.

In Their Own Words

Susan's story shows how the path to conception is both a mind and body endeavor. While Susan worked with several alternative modalities to prepare her body, she also worked with hypnosis to process the emotions that were at the root of her struggle with infertility. In the end, the in vitro procedure she had scheduled wasn't necessary. By creating a state of mind-body balance, Susan was able to conceive naturally.

Susan's Story
Using Complementary Modalities for Fertility

My husband and I started trying to get pregnant in January 2003 when I was almost thirty-five years old. I knew that thirty-five was the age in which fertility started to decline, so I had done everything I knew of to prepare for conception, planning to beat the odds. I had been off birth control pills for over a year, had read the books about preparing my body to get pregnant, and had followed the books' suggestions. I had also quit my high-stress job in order to facilitate conception and to be ready for my pregnancy and life as a stay-at-home mom, which I felt was surely only a few months away. Was I wrong! The journey had just begun.

By August 2003 I was still not pregnant, and I had started to become very frustrated and emotional every month when I got my period. So, in September 2003 we took the first step of going to a reproductive endocrinologist. I had already read the fertility books and thought that whatever problem I had could simply be fixed by some sort of pill. Once again, I was wrong. I went in for an HSG, and during the test I immediately felt a sharp pain on one side. The doctor looked at the monitor and told me that my tube on one side was blocked. I was stunned; something was wrong with me! And it was causing me problems in fulfilling my dream, a baby. Not only that, but now my husband was having problems fulfilling his dream too. "What would he think of me?" I thought. "What did I do to cause this blockage?" I was now really depressed.

My depression was replaced by hope, though, when our doctor explained that an IUI procedure could help me conceive even though one side was blocked. "Here was our solution," I thought! We did three IUI procedures with Clomid with no success. Once again my emotions were all over the place, exacerbated by the medication. Our doctor said this was the solution, but why wasn't it working? What would we do if this never worked? How long could we go on like this? I had come to the point where I realized that I needed additional help in handling our situation. My husband was very supportive and never blamed me for having a blocked tube, but I knew by now that there were many other options available to me. I was a believer in alternative therapies and professional counseling in conjunction with Western medicine, so my journey continued.

I started with acupuncture. Once again, I hung my hat on this procedure to be the solution. I had heard of many women who had acupuncture and then conceived. By the time I completed several sessions of acupuncture, though, I had heard of another modality for use in assisting fertility called uterine massage. Was that *the* solution? Having completed the acupuncture protocol for fertility suggested by my acupuncturist, I moved on to uterine massage. After meeting with the practitioner, I was once again filled with hope. She was so helpful and supportive! She had suggestions for my treatment that included dealing with my emotional health, which by now had completely deteriorated. Additionally, we planned to work on the positioning of my uterus which was tipped backward, a position that sometimes prevents conception. My practitioner also worked on my emotional support system and uterine massage in conjunction with my laparoscopy (designed to stop my blocked fallopian tube from leaking fluid and preventing implantation), and my next two unsuccessful IUI treatments with injectable medicine.

By this time, it was the fall of 2004, and I was now really beginning to see a connection between all the types of therapies I had used. Maybe there wasn't just one solution, I thought. I also could tell that although I was getting a lot of emotional help in my sessions for uterine massage, I needed another outlet for my feelings. I had participated in counseling several years back for help in handling a difficult childhood and believed in the power

of therapy. A support group suggested hypnotherapy as a resource for accessing deep-rooted feelings that can sometimes
prevent conception. It seemed to all be coming together. I had
been on a journey that included medical procedures to assist in
the physical process of conception, alternative therapy to
strengthen and prepare the body for conception, and now hypnotherapy to repair the mind and emotions.

I participated in hypnotherapy once a week for a few months
and made an incredible amount of progress. I could see the importance of every type of treatment I had been through and felt
positive once again.

I believe that the process of hypnotherapy helped me to unlock painful feelings that had been trapped inside my body for a
long time. I believe that holding these emotions inside my body
created an unhealthy state of being and resulted in a lot of tension. This tension may have contributed to my body's unwilling-
ness to conceive.

I feel that I had two emotional blocks to overcome in order to
conceive. The first emotional block was in regard to my struggle
with self-confidence. I grew up in a family in which perfection
seemed to be expected. Nothing I ever did seemed to be good
enough. This is a tough battle to fight because it never ends. The
question of whether or not one is being perfect stays with a person all day throughout every decision unless a person chooses
not to engage in this negative self-talk.

I also had an emotional block regarding my family of origin. I
felt a lot of sadness regarding the fact that my family of origin
created a difficult environment rather than a loving, nurturing
environment. I didn't believe that I would repeat this pattern
with my own child because I had been through previous counseling and had identified the negative patterns of my family.
However, I think I always had the question, *"What if* I did repeat
these patterns with my own child without intending to do so?" I
couldn't bear to think of myself inflicting that on my own child.

It was important, using mind-body work, that I was able to reach a feeling of closure with these issues.

In February 2005, my husband and I traveled to Hawaii. This trip was important because we had been on quite a journey and needed some time to reconnect with each other as well as some relaxation time before we geared up for a difficult IVF procedure. A few weeks following a fabulous trip, my husband suggested we "try one more time before the in vitro." Hesitantly, I agreed, not thinking too much about it and focusing my thoughts on the upcoming appointments we had scheduled for IVF. Finally, a few days before my period was scheduled to arrive, I took an early pregnancy test as I had done so many months before. I was planning to see the negative result and call the doctor's office for the first steps to our in vitro procedure. I wasn't prepared for what I found. The test was positive! I couldn't believe it. I was pregnant naturally after everything we had been through! It was March of 2005, and on November 21, 2005, our healthy baby girl was born.

My husband and I were on an incredible journey. It was a step-by-step process of healing my body and mind in such a way that they could perform a miracle, conception. There wasn't just one solution that provided the magic cure. Instead, each treatment was beneficial in its own way and led to another type of treatment that was also beneficial. In the end, it was all worth it. Our little girl is the joy of our life, and I became a better person and therefore a better mother.

WORKS CITED

1. Christiane Northrup, *Women's Bodies, Women's Wisdom* (New York, New York: Bantam Books, 1998), 418.

2. Suzy Greaves, "Can Hypnosis Help to Make You Pregnant?" *The Times Newspapers* (TimesOnLine.com), Mar. 5, 2002.

3. Andrew Weil, *Spontaneous Healing* (New York, New York: Fawcett Columbine, 1995), 134.

4. Deepak Copra, *Perfect Health: The Complete Mind Body Guide* (New York, Harmony Books, 1991), 12.

5. Ibid., 10.

6. Northrup, "Women's Bodies," 418.

CHAPTER SIX

THE DYNAMIC OF FEAR:

How the Past Can Affect the Present

One of the most common and powerful emotional blocks that can be trapped in our bodies is fear. We all know that fear and anxiety can become a part of one's make-up if that individual is subjected to traumatic experiences such as physical abuse, sexual abuse, or rape. People don't realize that fear can also develop from more subtle situations: a controlling parent can make a child so afraid of making a mistake or doing anything wrong that, as a result, the child learns to be fearful on a continual basis. That anxiety can take different forms when that child becomes an adult: for example, it can show up as low self-esteem or difficulty in completing tasks. While those two characteristics don't appear to be related to fear, one is driven by a fear of inadequacy while the other is driven by a fear of failure.

As I mentioned in chapter three, people commonly make false assumptions about their stress, attributing it to present-day conflicts and failing to acknowledge how their past issues are, in reality, a major contributor to what they are experiencing. Issues—such as anger, control, frustration, anxiety, and stress—are almost always generated and triggered by deep-seated fears. An issue such as anger is a perfect example of this. A woman's anger often has its beginnings when the woman is very young. Her anger might have grown out of constantly receiving criticism from her parents. She might find herself feeling as if whatever she did wasn't good enough. Those feelings of inadequacy will usually lead her to make sure that she excels at everything so that her parents won't have the opportunity to criticize her. That leads her to start trying to control everything in her life. When something goes wrong—and she feels that she could become the target of criticism—she gets angry. So, she attempts to always be in control, and when situations or individuals let her down, the anger emerges. The question then becomes, what is really at the root of the anger that is being expressed. Is she truly mad, or is she *afraid* of making a mistake: *afraid* that any mistake in her life will bring criticism; *afraid* that if there is a mistake, she is, once again, failing to measure up, not only to the standards of her parents but to the standards she has set for herself? Is this anger or is this really about fear: fear of failure, fear of inadequacy, or fear of not being perfect? After all, now that she is an adult, the people responsible for the anger, her parents, are probably out of the immediate picture and completely removed from the daily situations that are generating her anger.

The point is that people commonly associate their physical and emotional disharmonies with stress, and are unaware that the bigger issue is their fear. As I use a process called *age regression* (described in detail in chapter seven), where the client, in hypnosis, goes back to earlier times in their life, I have found that day-to-day pressure makes up a small portion of their stress, but the old embedded fears create the lion's share of their tension. Therefore, we do have to address stress from present-day situations. It is important to keep in mind, however, that the majority of our anxiety is probably related to our past, and our past is always affecting how we live our lives in the present.

This means that the common approach to working with infertility where the focus is strictly on what is happening in our present existence may be misguided. A woman can change her diet, eliminate drinking coffee and alcohol, carefully chart her cycles, and go to her doctor for follicle-stimulating drugs, but none of those things address the mental and emotional aspects of infertility. None of those changes are geared to reduce her stress, and, as I explained in the stress response chapter, there are several ways that stress impacts our physiology, creating infertile situations. Because of the way the physical body responds to stress, it is the number one contributor to infertility regardless of its source, and much of our stress comes directly from the fears that are stored in the subconscious mind.

To illustrate how fear can become a driving force that controls our present behavior, let's use an analogy of how the mind's programming can be similar to the inner workings of a computer. The material in the subconscious mind is often referred to as "programming," because that is exactly how it affects us. It programs our lives in much the same way that software programs control all of the functions, operations, and outcomes that can be performed on a computer. A woman can sit down at her "mental computer" and type in "I want to have a baby," and the response on the computer screen might read: "Sorry, that is not possible." She might ask the computer program again, and once more the answer coming from the software that holds the subconscious programming is: "Sorry, that is not possible." No matter how many times she enters her request, the response from the computer program is the same because that subconscious data is controlling the only possible output at that time.

If that woman had the ability to go into the software and look at the actual written program in her subconscious computer, she might find some very revealing information. It is somewhat like keeping a journal where of all of the experiences that had a profound effect on her life and behavior have been stored. An abbreviated version of her computer program—which has been recording all of her most significant life events—might look something like this:

Age	Fear	Subconscious Entry
4	Medical	Went to the hospital with broken arm. Incredible pain. Never want to have anything to do with medical procedures or hospitals again. Very scary!
5	Inadequacy, Abandonment	Parents divorced. It must be something I've done. I must not be lovable. My father left. I miss my father. Maybe if I am really good my mom will love me again.
6	Abandonment, Medical	Grandfather died after we visited him in the hospital. Also saw a woman there who was in lots of pain. I am afraid of doctors and hospitals. Why did Grandfather have to die?

Age	Fear	Subconscious Entry
8	Abandonment	My best friend moved away today. I'm sad because I'm afraid I'll never see her again.
9	Inadequacy, Imperfection, Failure	I broke one of my mom's dishes and she called me "stupid." I started to cry and she told me to grow up. I've got to be super careful from now on so that I never do anything wrong around her again.
12	Inadequacy, Betrayal	I had to give a speech in class and forgot what I was supposed to say. The other kids made fun of me, and I got a bad grade. I feel really stupid. Even my friends laughed at me.
18	Inadequacy, Betrayal	I caught my boyfriend going out with another girl. I really thought he loved me. I feel like such an idiot that I never figured this out.
24	Medical	Had surgery for endometriosis. It was horrible. I was extremely scared. The doctor said something about how I might have trouble getting pregnant if I ever want kids.
28	Inadequacy, Betrayal	My fiancé left me a note today saying that our relationship is over. I can't believe this is happening again. This is the third boyfriend that has left me. I can't trust anyone anymore.
32	Repeating Family Dysfunction, Failure	Got married today. This was supposed to be a happy day, but my mother refused to go to the ceremony because my father was there. I am so fed up with family stuff. There has been nothing but arguing and fighting in my family since the day I was born. What if my marriage ends up like that?

If this list represents a part of the program that is written into a woman's subconscious computer, it is easy to see some of the ways that her programming is not receptive to getting pregnant. Here are some of the issues that might arise out of those events and how those issues could be interfering with her ability to have a baby:

- There are fears around doctors, hospitals, and medical procedures. If she decides to use ART, her body and cells may be resistant. (See chapter eight on cellular reprogramming.) If she gets pregnant naturally, she might still have extreme fears around check-ups and childbirth, creating lots of biological stress.

- There appears to be little confidence in the family unit. She witnessed much fighting and arguing and a failed relationship with her parents. She may have concerns that she could repeat some of those same dysfunctions.

- She might have a difficult time with abandonment, betrayal, and feeling unsupported. There has been a pattern where she loses the people—her father, best friend, grandfather, and boyfriends—who have been close to her. Based on this repeating pattern, there could be a subconscious fear that if she got pregnant, her husband might leave as well.

- The patterns of inadequacy will likely affect her confidence. In several events, she felt or was called "stupid." She may doubt whether she can get pregnant, whether she deserves to get pregnant, or whether she would be a good mother.

- The doctor suggested that she may have a difficult time having children. Since he is a person of authority, her subconscious might embrace this belief making it her truth.

- Her resolve to never make a mistake or let people down can easily become tied to her efforts to get pregnant. She may be determined that she is *not* going to let everyone down: she is going to *make sure* that she gets pregnant so as to not disappoint the people in her life. When a woman takes that position, she puts a great deal of pressure on herself. That pressure becomes stress, and stress is a major block to fertility.

Keep in mind that this is *not* a conscious process. A woman doesn't tell herself to register these specific decisions and experiences into her subconscious mind; instead, it is a subtle process where the mind grabs onto the information that it feels is relevant in each situation. At the time, she may only know that she is undergoing an emotional event and has no idea what kind of programming actually becomes part of her subconscious make-up.

The information in the subconscious computer programming is much more complex and detailed than the example given here; however, that doesn't mean that we have to process every single issue we've encountered in our life in order to get pregnant. Instead, there are usually two to four issues that present themselves as what I call *themes*—issues that are recurring and carry more weight—and it is those themes that can create the major blocks. In the case above, the medical fears and feelings of inadequacy might be the themes that are creating huge barriers to conception, while the concern about repeating the dysfunctional family dynamics might not be an issue at all. The point is that everything in our past goes into the subconscious mind, and those emotional events and issues profoundly affect fertility. Getting pregnant isn't as simple as looking at the current, everyday stuff.

To further illustrate how our subconscious programming is the principal driving force in how we feel, react, and behave in different situations, we can look at another example: a case of being around an individual who has had too much to drink. For most people this instantly generates uncomfortable feelings due to the drunken behavior. This response—which is very common—is most often triggered by the subconscious programming. It isn't the conscious mind that brings up the discomfort; those feelings are generated from the subconscious. The reaction may be triggered by memories of a friend or family member who drank too much and was abusive, or became emotionally unavailable, or created situations where they lost control and hurt themselves, or became a very different person when they were under the influence of alcohol. Our rational mind might tell us that our reaction to the drunken individual is illogical because those days with the drunken family member are long gone, but the critical mind is not in charge and therefore the reaction occurs whether we like it or not. The feelings of fear or discomfort are coming from the subconscious mind. It is as if our critical mind is saying "don't be scared," or "don't let it bother you," while our gut feeling—coming from the subconscious—is being overpowered with fear and anxiety.

In the same way, our bodies and psyche are constantly reacting to emotional triggers that affect fertility. Instead of a drunken individual bringing up feelings of fear, it can be any one of a number of daily triggers that generate a negative response in the physical body, and those responses impact the ability to conceive. In the earlier example regarding the woman with the subconscious computer, perhaps every time she thinks about childbirth, her body reacts with an uncomfortable, fearful feeling about hospitals and medical procedures. Perhaps, whenever her husband goes out of town on a business trip, a part of her starts to fear that he may not come back, bringing up feelings of abandonment. Perhaps, whenever she makes a mistake, she gets upset with herself and resolves that she can prove her worthiness by getting pregnant and having great kids. A moment later, when she remembers that she is struggling with infertility, she might feel an overwhelming sense of sadness, defeat, and pressure to perform. The point is that these responses are occurring on a regular basis—usually at a deep level that is often overlooked by our conscious awareness—and these old issues are triggering responses that affect our physiology and ability to conceive. The response in the body—whether it is reacting to fear, sadness, inadequacy, or any one of a number of emotions—may stimulate the production of cortisol, upset the hormones related to fertility, reduce the blood flow to the uterus by constricting the blood vessels or other physiological responses that are detrimental to fertility.

The pattern is commonplace, and it affects all of us, every day of our lives:

Environmental Trigger
↓
Subconscious Emotional Response
↓
Physical Response

The physical response or final outcome is almost always a stress response, and stress responses are what create infertility. (See chapter four regarding stress reduction for a more detailed explanation of the physical stress responses that are detrimental to reproduction.) If our programming brings up feelings of sadness, anger, fear, inadequacy, or any one of a number of emotions, we might be able to consciously block or ignore that feeling in order to maintain an even demeanor in public, but it doesn't mean that our physical body is able to avoid the corresponding physical response triggered by that emotion.

A closer look at the issues and events that were written into the subconscious software of the woman in the example above reveals how fear can have a huge impact on our lives and our ability to conceive. Every issue on the list is in some way rooted in fear. There is fear of medical procedures, hospitals, doctors, fear that her doctor's diagnosis (at age twenty-four) might come true, abandonment, repeating dysfunctional family dynamics, betrayal, being imperfect or inadequate, and the fear of failure. *The fact is that most of our issues are in some way based in fear.*

PROGRAMMING THE SUBCONSCIOUS MIND

Our subconscious is continually recording information. However, certain situations can enhance or increase the impact of the new material and give it more power and control over how we feel and behave. There are three circumstances in which information can become deeply ingrained in our programming:

1. When the information is introduced during the early years of childhood.
2. When we hear something said by a person of authority.
3. When we witness or experience a traumatic event.

Our subconscious mind is most vulnerable when it is subjected to these three sets of circumstances. Information introduced during those critical times packs the most powerful punch.

A CHILD IS AN OPEN BOOK

Remember the old children's saying: "Sticks and stones may break my bones, but words will never hurt me." Maybe an asterisk should be attached to that with fine print that reads: "except when it comes to young children." When we are young, negative words and images that may seem powerless at the time can evolve into obsessive impressions that make it almost impossible to have a positive belief system about many of life's challenges, including pregnancy.

It is said that a child is like an open book because a child is recording everything that occurs—with very little filtering—in his or her world. During the early part of childhood—especially up to the time when we turn six—our subconscious is wide open and absorbing everything we observe around us. At this early age, the conscious or critical mind has not sufficiently matured enough to act as a filter and hasn't developed the capability to discriminate between what is truth and what information can be rejected.

When a child continually hears statements like, "you're so stupid," or "can't you do anything right," or "why can't you be like your sister," the message is very clear: this child has been programmed to *know* that she is inadequate. In all of these situations, she is being told that she's not good enough. A child doesn't need to hear this very often for this to become part of her belief system. In cases where a parent is full of passion or rage when one of these comments is voiced, it can magnify the power of the message tenfold. Ironically, many parents will say these things under the assumption that the child will perform at a higher standard. Instead, it is more likely to make the child feel that they can't do anything right and so they perform poorly in many tasks due to their lack of self-confidence. Statements that are continually repeated create the strongest imprints in the subconscious mind because of the reinforcement.

As a child gets older, the subconscious tape recorder is able to be more selective about what is recorded, and it develops the capability of filtering some of the information that it is exposed to: the conscious mind will start to step in and discriminate between what we hold to be true, and what might be information that can be disregarded. However, words or events that are *emotionally* charged carry a lot of weight and can still leave a powerful imprint. For example, when a teacher makes it clear that one of her students is the only one in the class who isn't able to grasp a concept or perform a certain task, it is likely that the student will never forget that moment of extreme embarrassment. Or, a child who performs poorly in a piano recital or in a school play will probably continue to have difficulty when asked to speak or perform in front of a crowd because their subconscious mind has permanently recorded the anxiety that arose during the moment that they perceived as a complete disaster. The logical or conscious mind may have even forgotten the original event that is affecting the behavior, but the subconscious mind sends continual reminder messages in the form of anxiety or distress whenever they are called upon to stand in front of others.

As much as we'd like to believe that we get over or release all of this old, often dysfunctional programming when we turn eighteen and move out of the house, it doesn't work that way. It remains part of our subconscious programming, and much of that embedded information from childhood can become a negative force during the struggle with infertility.

Deep feelings of inadequacy, for example, can wreak havoc with the pregnancy process. This can manifest in a couple of different ways. One possibility is the woman who believes she may not be worthy or deserving of having children. This can be greatly compounded or reinforced if that woman has done something in her past—such as going through a time of promiscuity or having an abortion—because feelings of guilt from her past will reinforce her feelings of lack or unworthiness around having a baby.

The other, more common scenario, is the inadequacy felt by the woman who is possessed by high expectations or perfectionism. (See chapter seven, about perfectionism and expectations.) The tremendous drive of a woman with these characteristics can lead her to be determined to *not* let this one and only thing she hasn't been able to do in life get the best of her. Her determination, coupled with the fear of failure—a response to her feelings of inadequacy—is so strong that, on some level, she essentially becomes resolute in her actions to *make* this happen and thereby multiplies the tension and pressure she puts on herself. That pressure or stress is one of the biggest hindrances to fertility, and the outcome of that tension is that it makes her body much less likely to reproduce.

Oftentimes the drive, motivation and emotional components that originated in our childhood subconscious minds affect our behavior in ways that almost seem to be mysterious. It isn't coming from our *logical* source, and it often makes no sense to the adult critical mind, but something inside of us, from long ago, can be controlling the behavior, feelings, and reactions to our current situations.

WORDS FROM PEOPLE IN POSITIONS OF AUTHORITY

Words from people of authority carry incredible weight. In a sense, when these people talk, it can embed those words immediately into the subconscious. Doctors are one of the best examples of this. For instance, when a fertility specialist tells a woman, "You are too old to get pregnant with your own eggs," those words go directly into the subconscious mind. If those words are accepted by the subconscious—and they did come from a specialist—then it becomes almost impossible for this woman to have the confidence in her body to conceive unless she elects to use donor eggs. Her belief system also sends that message to her cells (see chapter eight, on cellular reprogramming), and instead of trying to overcome this new belief and create healthy follicles—through mind/body healing and alternative modalities—she will most likely go through a period of grieving and become acquiescent. Whatever chances she may have had to become pregnant naturally may have just been reduced to zero if she accepts this new authoritative programming.

Another common occurrence is when a sixteen-year-old girl has a gynecological issue such as an ovarian cyst removed and the doctor says, "You might have trouble getting pregnant when you are older." Those words are never forgotten. The weight of these words is incredibly powerful because not only were they spoken at a traumatic time and by an authority figure, but also because the young adult mind, as mentioned earlier, is still more open and vulnerable. This information may now become her *truth* and subsequently a powerful block to fertility.

Another message from an authority figure might come from a mother who, for the most part, has been a good role model for her daughter, and then in one angry moment loses her temper and screams at her twelve-year-old: "You just wait 'til you get older. You'll never be a good mother." No parent can be perfect, and these moments are going to happen. It's inevitable. The point is that this message can be permanently lodged into the daughter's subconscious mind. Again, coming from an authority figure, this kind of communication when received by a child carries twice the power. While that event and the words spoken might be forgotten by the conscious mind, there is something deep inside of that woman when she becomes an adult that might question if she really can be a good mother. It is another subtle way that the subconscious communicates through messages that won't go away until we reprogram them.

TRAUMATIC EVENTS

Witnessing or being part of a traumatic event can also leave images burned into the subconscious. For example, a woman, or young girl, who is witness to a traumatic childbirth may be recording that information at a very deep level. She might walk away from that experience with newly embedded fears about what might happen to her if she were to ever get pregnant and have to give birth.

Another example might occur in a family where one of the children has a serious emotional or physical challenge. The siblings of that child might observe the behaviors and decide that the same scenario might play out for them if they were to have children. Somewhere, deep inside, a decision is made that they don't want to repeat this dynamic. Sometimes it turns into a fear of having children, and that fear has the potential to escalate into a powerful, subconscious block.

Families where alcoholism, drug use, or abuse is present may create fertility blocks because that woman who wants to get pregnant has subconscious concerns about what she has experienced or observed. Could the situation arise again if she has kids? Could her child be subjected to this same behavior from one of her family members? Could that behavior be repeated by her husband or even herself? Perhaps as a teen she witnessed an event triggered by her father's explosive temper and occasionally she has noticed that her husband can also become angry. Her husband's anger may be one-twentieth of what she witnessed from her father, but that little bit is enough to tap into the doubts and fears she has about having children. Could that escalate? Could her children be subjected to what she witnessed when her father lost control? It was a traumatic event that is still very real in her subconscious mind. It is also that doubt or fear that triggers a physical stress response in her body. It may have the potential to affect her mind and body during every cycle until that belief is identified and those feelings are released.

HOW TO OVERCOME THE PAST

In order to release what has built up in the past, the old programming, whether it is words or beliefs, has to be addressed, stripped of its power and replaced by positive beliefs. How does that happen? The first course of action is uncovering or identifying what is programmed or hidden in the depths of the subconscious mind. After uncovering the beliefs and emotions, the next step is to process and heal those old ideas and issues. The third step is to plug in or create new beliefs to replace the old. (A more detailed example of this work is included in chapter thirteen.)

For example, the woman mentioned earlier in this chapter who at age sixteen had the ovarian cyst removed, may need to *imagine* going back and comforting her younger self during the operation. She may need to unplug the belief that this operation permanently affected her fertility: even if it was problematic for one ovary, the subconscious may need to be reminded that the other ovary is perfectly operational. She might also need to replace those fears of never having a child with a visualization where she sees herself pregnant and later imagines she is holding her baby (see chapter nine on meditation and visualization).

Some readers might think that common logic should tell her all of this, but it is a perfect illustration of how our subconscious minds and our fears are *not* governed by logic. The subconscious is often quite il-logical because it is based on feelings and beliefs and old memories that are created by emotions, *not analytic thought*. Logically, flying is safer than driving, but telling someone who is afraid of flying to be logical about getting on an airplane doesn't work because the fear that is gov-erning their behavior is coming from the *often illogical* subconscious mind. If using simple logic was an effective way of changing our sub-conscious programming, there would be no fear or doubt or anger or other issues because we could simply use rational thought to remove them. Unfortunately, it isn't that easy. There is work that has to be done.

The most efficient way to work with the subconscious—and the modality that is designed specifically to do this type of work—is hypno-sis. Hypnosis is designed to bypass the logical mind and directly address the subconscious material. It is safe and the client is *always* in control during the process. People who are afraid of hypnotherapy will find, as they do research, that what they've seen in movies and on TV is noth-ing like the actual experience. Hypnotherapy is a beneficial, healing modality that brings us back to our own power so that we can regain control over how we desire our lives to be. (See chapter thirteen to learn more about hypnotherapy.)

Those who would prefer to use other modalities may have difficulty achieving the same levels of success. Much of the subconscious infor-mation is so deeply buried that it might take five years of ordinary dia-logue to uncover it, and there is a good chance that much of it will never be revealed by trying to talk it out. Almost always, the issues need to be dealt with directly, which requires accessing the *emotions* con-nected to that issue. When the subconscious mind uncovers a signifi-cant belief, based on past programming, it is often accompanied by an emotional release, and this signals where the healing work must be done. Any modality that offers to heal the subconscious without ad-dressing the issues, or claims it can be done without processing the emotional responses, is unlikely to generate any lasting results.

In Their Own Words

Marilyn's account of her fertility journey includes several examples of how old programming from the past was affecting her present-day ability to conceive. Those old issues included two lost pregnancies, the doctor's diagnosis that she would need to use donor eggs (which was contrary to what she had always pictured when she was growing up), familial control issues, mental illness in the family, expectations from the birth family, feelings of inadequacy, and so on. It was important to process these sources of stress and negativity in order for Marilyn to prepare her body to be receptive for her in vitro procedure.

Marilyn's Story
Overcoming Family Expectations

We started out with four and a half years of not conceiving before going to see a fertility specialist. At that point, we started doing IUIs and had one successful pregnancy. When that ended prematurely, at the beginning of the second trimester, it was very devastating. Then, I had a second pregnancy not too long after that, which was lost as well. That's when we started to realize the problems were deeper than we originally thought. The doctor's diagnosis was that we needed to go the route of egg donation. That was another huge blow. I felt that all this information was overwhelming to me, and I needed some tools to sort through it and deal with it, and that's when I started hypnotherapy.

More and more unraveled as we went through our sessions. I began to realize all of the emotional thoughts and fears I had. Specifically, we had a lot of control issues in our family and a history of mental illness. I was afraid that I might be passing these things on to my children. Another emotional block I addressed in hypnotherapy was deeply ingrained expectations about how my family wanted me to be a professional. Their focus was not on us having children, it was for me to be successful in my career. I needed to come to terms with what their wants were, and what my desires were in life for my own destiny. Also, I needed to come to terms with saying I was worthy of whatever I wanted in life and that other expectations of me were not paramount to my life. The mind-body work helped me work through what were rational and irrational fears, and it helped me recognize situations where the emotional blocks that I had created were getting in the way of a successful pregnancy.

The hypnosis helped a lot with developing coping skills to help me come to terms with all the information coming at me. It seemed for me that it was one thing after another. Originally I thought I'd go in and have one IUI and have a baby. The holistic approach combining acupuncture with hypnotherapy and a support group helped me tackle it from all angles and enabled me to be in the best physical, mental, and spiritual place I could be. That way, when I did have a baby, I would have a healthy mental state and I would pass on good things to my children.

I found that learning how to do a daily meditation was critical for changing my belief system about myself and learning how to cope. When negative thoughts came up in my mind, I had tools to help dissipate them and regain control of my own thoughts instead of having other people's thoughts work their way into my brain. This work, and these life changes, started with fertility, but in every aspect of my life it has helped me gain that adult independence that I needed. I still use the tools I learned in hypnosis, to work on other areas of my life. It was a tremendous experience and a really important piece to getting where I wanted to be.

Through egg donation, I have twins who are two years old, wild and crazy and a part of my life that makes me very happy.

CHAPTER SEVEN

THE IMPERFECT WORLD
OF THE PERFECTIONIST

Someone recently asked me if there was a common characteristic or pattern that I've observed in clients who struggle with infertility. Without hesitation, I answered in one word: perfectionism. It seems paradoxical in our society today, where there are so many complaints about apathy and recklessness in the population, that perfectionism would appear to be a negative trait. After all, the corporate world loves these individuals and often lauds their dedicated work ethic. We rarely see anything written or hear much about the negative aspects of perfectionism, much less in conjunction with infertility, but the pressure within the overachiever is immense. It might be the most common reason why the infertility client is unsuccessful in what they want to accomplish. It is the one quality that I've observed in about three quarters of the women who have trouble conceiving. So, for those readers who get to this chapter and think, "I don't need to read this. It doesn't apply to me," read on—because perfectionism has an insidious way of controlling our lives without us ever being fully aware or acknowledging its presence.

How do we define or identify this quality in a person? It is difficult because perfectionism can take many different forms. The easy answer is that it is the high achiever, or the person who puts in lots of extra hours at work, or the person whose house is always immaculate, or the person who is very conscientious about their appearance, or the person who is extremely hard on themselves when they make a mistake. Despite the obvious manifestations of perfectionism, oftentimes that person also has an area of non-perfection in their life so that the overachiever can deny that perfectionism applies to them. In other words, the person who keeps the immaculate house might tell you that they are terrible in social situations, thus providing *proof* that they do have their faults.

In general, the perfectionist tries to control the situations and outcomes of everything around them in order to ensure that there is no failure or disappointment in their life. Control is a key component of perfectionism. It starts with self-control and then escalates into attempting to control elements of the world around them. People will often admit they are controlling or they have very high expectations of themselves, but they rarely consider that they might be a *perfectionist*. It may be a matter of semantics. The word "perfectionist" has a somewhat negative connotation in our society. It sounds a little too extreme even for those who admit they are controlling or have high expectations of themselves.

In relation to infertility, many women who are trying to conceive are often trying to control the process down to some of the smallest details. They may say, "I've been able to accomplish everything I set out to do in life until now," making a reference to their inability to get pregnant. In many instances, one word could be changed in that statement to ascertain the real truth: "I've been able to *control* everything I set out to do in life until now." I always tell women during the first session, "The more you try to control the conception process, the farther you push it away."

The perfection cycle usually begins early in life with high expectations. These may grow out of the relationships with the birth family. Many times, the child is not getting the love or acknowledgment that they need, and feel like they must somehow prove they are worthy. That drive escalates over the years. It doesn't go away when the child leaves home and starts to live on their own. What emerges is an adult who will do whatever they can to ensure that outcomes are always positive. In other words, they try to control the people and events around them to avoid any kind of failure. If there is a failure, they are often relentless about beating themselves up. To sum it up, they are trying to make sure that everything is *perfect*.

Perfectionists are individuals who live their lives operating with extremely high expectations for themselves, and sometimes also the people around them. In the biology of the perfectionist, the sympathetic nervous system is turned on all the time: they feel like they are constantly under pressure to perform. When they fail, they are devastated, and it is very difficult for them to practice self-forgiveness.

It is important to look at how this becomes a part of one's make-up and how this characteristic affects infertility.

THE ORIGINS OF PERFECTIONISM

As I mentioned earlier, perfectionism usually grows out of expectations that are introduced in childhood, and it often originates as a result or outcome of the relationship that children have with their parents. The family dynamics can be varied, but the end result is the same: the child emerges with such high expectations of how they are to perform in life that there is no alternative but to be perfect.

Here are some of the common family dynamics that I believe can produce a child with extraordinarily high expectations:

- Families that push to over achieve. They want their kids to be the best at everything.

- Families where image and appearance mean everything. These families are concerned with what people might say or what the neighbors might think.

- Families where a child feels that one of his or her siblings is the favorite, so the rejected child—as they see themselves—has to prove their worthiness. That child wants the same level of love and acceptance as their sibling so they operate under the assumption that if they perform every task at a high level, they will get equal recognition and love.

- Families where there is neglect and a child feels they have to excel in order to get love, attention, or acknowledgment from their parents. Neglect can be the physical absence of one or both parents.

It can also occur if a child feels an emotional distancing or disconnect coming from one or both parents.

- Families where expectations are never stated, but understood: it is understood that you will get A's in school. This child may not receive accolades for their achievements, but if their performance is even slightly sub par, the disappointment expressed by their parents is very clear.

- Families where love is withheld in order to control or manipulate a child's behavior. The child keeps trying harder in hopes of getting the parents' approval, under the assumption that being perfect will win their love. Sometimes these parents are emotionally incapable of expressing love or they withhold that love realizing that they have found a way of shaping the child's behavior so that the child never does anything wrong.

THE PATHS OF PERFECTIONISM

When the child grows up with any of these family dynamics, I believe that the pressure from the expectations will lead them to take one of three paths. The numbers and descriptions below are based on observations and client histories I have assimilated and recorded over the years in my practice:

1. The *pure perfectionist* tries to control everything in their lives so there can be no negative outcomes. About 10 percent of the children who grow up in perfectionist families fall into this category. These are the people who come right out and admit that they are perfectionists.

2. The *rebel*. All this person knows and understands is that they can't live up to the high expectations imposed by the family or themselves. It is too much pressure for them to attempt to meet these expectations. In a sense, they stop trying and are crippled by the fear of failure. These are the ones who have given up. They rarely finish college, take jobs that are considered beneath their potential and choose partners who are well below the standards set by

the family. People in this group often turn to drugs and alcohol. This comprises about 20 percent of the children who grow up in perfectionist families.

It is extremely rare for them to seek out a therapist because, if they solve their problems, then they will have the burden of living up to their expectations. They usually have parents or siblings who are dedicated to *fixing* them, an objective that will never come to fruition.

3. The *hybrid* is a combination of the two paths described above. This person is about 90 percent perfectionist and about 10 percent rebel. Most of what they do is performed at a very high level, but they try to deny the perfection and control by having a few selected areas of rebellion. An example of the hybrid is the person who will boast that they do exceptional work at the office and then follow that with, "but you should see my house: it's a mess." The rebellion—often a reaction to their upbringing—is their way of trying to prove that they aren't a perfectionist. Sometimes they don't want to acknowledge it. Oftentimes, they aren't aware that their life is governed by high expectations. The remaining 70 percent of children who grow up in families with high expectations seem to fall into this category.

Many people don't know or won't willingly accept that they are perfectionists if they fall into the *hybrid* category. It provides an opportunity for them to either rebel enough to deny it or be completely unaware that it applies to them.

Interestingly enough, a perfectionist family with several children will often have children in all three of these categories, each expressing the pressures of high expectations in their own way.

POSSIBLE ORIGINS OF PERFECTIONISM

Based on the events over the past hundred years—the Great Depression, large numbers of immigrant families struggling to survive, rationing during the World Wars—it makes sense that high expectations have emerged as a dominant quality in many families. Not only was there pressure to compete for simple survival, but the twentieth century was also considered an opportunistic time for hard-working individuals to move up to higher socioeconomic classes.

One might argue that today's fertility client is two or more generations removed from those world-changing events. How could those events impact her? It appears that high expectations are often passed from one generation to the next. Sometimes the pressure to overachieve is clearly defined by what the parents expect from their children, but it is also quite common for this behavior to be adopted by a child who is watching as that behavior is modeled by one or both of their parents.

So, the immigrant family that "worked their fingers to the bone" modeled that quality for their children, who struggled to survive during the post-Depression era. They, in turn, passed that work ethic on to their children who faced challenges at colleges and universities, and a corporate world that can often be discriminatory, competitive, and ruthless. The pressure and competition may be different for each generation, but they all believe that they can face their challenges by relying on the determination they learned from their parents.

PERFECTIONISM AND INFERTILITY

The negative effects of perfectionism are especially evident in the infertility client as she does everything in her power to try to create a positive outcome. She has read all the books, meticulously charted her cycles, made lifestyle changes based on articles she has read, scoured the internet for information, carefully scheduled her lovemaking, and is still left feeling frustrated and inadequate by the inability to achieve her goal. Despite these determined efforts to *control* this process, all of this conscious thinking and doing is actually creating a barrier between her desire and her fertility because of the incredible stress that comes with pushing herself to achieve the perfect outcome. This internal stress or pressure from continually trying to meet high expectations is not conducive to good physical or emotional health. As stated earlier, the sympathetic nervous system of someone under this kind of stress is *always* switched on, which greatly diminishes the body's ability to conceive. It also generates a high level of tension in the body that often goes unnoticed or feels normal because it has been present her entire life. The body of the perfectionist isn't relaxed enough for the hypothalamus gland—the brain's control center for reproductive activity—to function correctly. This, in turn, can upset the balance of hormones and the body's ability to conceive. The uterus isn't relaxed enough for adequate blood flow and is not a receptive environment for the embryo to implant. The cumulative effect of a lifetime of continually pushing to meet high expectations creates a stress level so great that the mind and body can no longer work in harmony to support conception. It is an expectations/perfectionism/control cycle that makes conception and full-term pregnancy almost impossible.

DENIAL OR LACK OF AWARENESS

Most perfectionists will initially be unaware or unwilling to admit that this characteristic applies to them. Remember, only 10 percent, the *pure perfectionists*, are going to admit it. The *hybrid* perfectionist has enough rebel in them that they will deny it or simply not believe it applies to them. Even after reading this chapter, people will admit to the expectations and control, but that is probably where the admissions will end. That word "perfectionist" is too hard for many to embrace.

THE PERFECTIONISM QUIZ

This quiz is designed to help identify behaviors and characteristics of the perfectionist personality. Since the goal of this work is to better understand the blocks to fertility, it is important to make an honest assessment so that changes can be made to lessen the pressure we feel from high expectations and increase the likelihood of conception.

I recommend that you take this quiz with your partner or a friend. As you evaluate yourself, they will also evaluate you. It is important to listen to their input because this is one of those cases where someone on the outside can sometimes be more honest than we can be with ourselves.

Answer each of the following questions with a number value of 3, 2, 1, or 0, depending on how strongly that question characterizes you and your habits. .

3 = Always applies to me.

2 = Sometimes applies to me.

1 = Rarely applies to me

0 = Never applies to me.

_____ 1. Do you keep a "to do" list at work or at home?

_____ 2. Does it upset you when people don't follow the rules (i.e, co-workers, other drivers)?

_____ 3. Do you tend to put off "fun activities" (a fun activity *does not* include your workout or exercise routine) until the work is done?

_____ 4. Do you feel like you are always busy doing things and rarely give yourself an *hour or two* for relaxation (again, exercise or a workout is not considered relaxation)?

_____ 5. Do you find yourself saying (about co-workers, businesses, construction/repair people) that you just expect them to do their job correctly?

_____ 6. Do you clean your house or apartment at least once a week?

_____ 7. Do you feel—or have people told you—that you are controlling?

_____ 8. Do you work more than forty hours a week?

_____ 9. Do you make the bed every day?

_____ 10. Are the dishes done before you go to bed at least 95 percent of the time?

_____ 11. Do you double-check for mistakes (such as grammar and spelling errors) more than once before you send an e-mail or electronic communication?

_____ 12. Did you grow up with parents who had high expectations of you?

_____ 13. Was your birth family worried about what other people would think or say?

_____ 14. Did you have a sibling who seemed to get more attention (whether it was good or bad attention) than you?

_____ 15. Is your body weight either under or within five pounds of what the height/weight charts say you should be?

_____ 16. Do you exercise more than four days a week?

_____ 17. On weekdays, do you always make sure you have make-up on and are dressed nicely before you leave the house?

_____ 18. In your lifetime, have there been occasions where you made up your mind to "show them" or prove yourself?

_____ 19. Are you tough on yourself when you make a mistake?

_____ 20. Do you find that there is never enough time in the day because you are constantly going or doing?

_____ 21. Do you consider yourself to be a type A or driven personality?

_____ 22. Do you get very uncomfortable when you are late for a meeting or appointment?

_____ 23. Do you ever find yourself wanting to succeed at a task or accomplishment in order to impress your parents, a rival, or a friend?

_____ 24. Do you sometimes feel guilty or think about things you should be doing when you are supposed to be having fun?

_____ 25. Do you consider a day to be a good day if you were able to get a lot of things accomplished?

_____ Total

_____ Total score evaluation by your friend

GRADING SCALE

75–56. You might be used to being in the top percentile. This score suggests that you are a perfectionist. It is an indication that perfectionism and stress reduction should be two key areas of focus in your fertility work.

55–40. This score suggests that you might have some tendencies toward perfectionism. If your friend or partner has a similar score for you, then it is an area to watch to make sure that control and expectations don't become overpowering. If your partner gave you a much higher score than you gave yourself, that indicates there might be some degree of denial on your part.

39–below. A score in this range—provided it is in agreement with the total given to you by your partner—means that you are not one who falls into the perfectionist category.

STRATEGIES FOR SUCCESS

Clinically, the best way to explore whether or not someone is a perfectionist is by using hypnotic age regression. Age regression is a technique where a client, while in hypnosis, goes back to experiences that occurred earlier in life. It is often helpful to allow the client to observe what they were feeling and experiencing and how they were reacting when they were in a specific setting or situation in their past. For example, a woman may return to a classroom setting when she was in elementary school. If she reports that her body is extremely tense and full of fear because she is afraid of making a mistake and getting a bad grade, that may be an indication that she is feeling pressure from high expectations. If the client has a different reaction—such as feeling like she doesn't fit in and none of the other students like her—then that response may indicate a different issue might apply, such as feelings of inadequacy. Unlike trying to *consciously remember* old times where the memories and details are often quite vague, in hypnotic age regression the feelings and thought processes from those old experiences emerge very clearly *from the subconscious mind*, and it is that information that reveals what issues were relevant at that time and may still be a factor in our present life. The other advantage of using hypnosis to access the subconscious material is that the memories stored there will usually take the person directly to the scenes that played a major role in creating or establishing the significant issues which are still driving current attitudes and behaviors. In other words, the subconscious mind often goes straight to the scenes and experiences where the healing needs to take place. Conversely, if one simply attempts to *consciously remember* scenes that might be important in their life, the critical factor will usually block most of the relevant scenes and keep those issues buried in the subconscious. Conscious remembering is a very slow process that rarely reveals the concerns or the pertinent emotions that need to be addressed.

If the client returns to three or four different scenes from the past, they can easily make their own observations about the level of tension in their body at various ages and make their own assessment as to whether or not perfectionism has been a factor in their life. If perfectionism is present, the individual will clearly feel the stress in their body that accompanies high expectations. Since this characteristic is embedded in the programming of the subconscious mind, this investigative process is necessary to provide a means whereby the client can discover their own level of perfection-driven stress. There is absolutely no point in asking the *conscious mind*: only 10 percent of these individuals are going to admit or understand that this trait applies to them.

Because this trait is usually established at an early age, perfectionism is very deeply programmed. The most important part of breaking the pattern is discovery, seeing how it impacts our behavior, and then applying tools for recovery. These patterns and beliefs can be overcome, and when that happens, the client can experience positive changes that open the door to fertility.

Some ways to work with the stress associated with perfectionism include stress reduction, meditation, forgiveness work, and incorporating strategies in daily life that help with releasing or letting go of obsessive tendencies. To clarify, the objective isn't to become complacent and stop executing at a competent level, but rather it is simply to become more comfortable with performing well as opposed to always pushing to excel.

In order to practice this, it is sometimes beneficial for an individual to take part in an activity where she can give herself permission to be imperfect, have fun, and experience self-love. (See the activity below.) Another tool or assignment is to have the perfectionist increase their awareness by keeping a record of every task where perfectionism starts to become a factor in influencing their behavior. Awareness is a powerful first step in generating change.

MEDITATIVE EXERCISE NUMBER ONE

What does being a perfectionist feel like? Take a minute and close your eyes. Take ten deep breaths, letting go of any stress or tension each time you exhale.

Imagine a time in your life where you were under incredible stress. Maybe there was a project that had to be finished at work or you had to do a speech in front of a group of people. Maybe there was a period in your life where you were consumed by feelings of being overwhelmed. Take an inventory of how you felt and what you experienced at that time in your life. How is your breathing? How is your heart rate? How does your stomach feel? Is there tightness in your muscles? Is your jaw tight or clenched? This is the kind of pressure that can be created with high expectations. Are these feelings common for you?

After you finish this exercise, imagine that you are in a beautiful place in nature. Take ten deep breaths. Breathe in calmness and serenity, and when you exhale, let go of any of the tension you brought up with this exercise. Breathe out the need to win or control or excel or look perfect in the eyes of anyone you may feel is judging you. Take a moment and love yourself unconditionally. After you have brought calmness into your body, you can open your eyes. It is often helpful to journal or discuss this with your partner.

MEDITATIVE EXERCISE NUMBER TWO

Close your eyes again. Take a few deep breaths.

Imagine going back to the last time you had *important* family or friends over to your house for a get-together or to stay at your house. How much effort did you put forth to make sure that everything was just right? How much time did you spend preparing? What was the extent of time that went into cleaning, preparing, cooking, testing menu ideas to know what to serve, yard work, home repairs, painting, carpet cleaning, shopping for food, shopping for clothes, shopping for household items such as new towels, haircuts, etc. When you have a clear idea of what was done to prepare, open your eyes and make up a list where you include *everything you remember doing or worrying about*. Assign a time value to each chore on the list.

The non-perfectionists might spend two to four hours to clean, run to the store, and prepare the meal. Perfectionists will take several hours—sometimes parts of several days—to prepare. This is another way for someone to get an idea of whether or not perfectionism applies to them.

PERFECTIONISM IN NON-FERTILITY APPLICATIONS

In addition to infertility, I have noticed that perfectionism may be at the root of other disharmonies affecting our bodies and emotions, and I believe the tremendous stress in the highly competitive overachiever is a major factor. Here are just a couple of those areas where it appears to be an issue.

If perfectionism is present and not addressed, any deviation from an individual's desired outcome can be a huge setback. For example, if a person with weight issues should falter and eat something that they had intended to give up on their diet, the perfectionist will often enter into a "who cares" mode. In other words, they will decide that since they have slipped up, they might as well eat anything they want because they have failed. For the perfectionist, it is all or nothing. When there is a breakdown, they have failed and it is very difficult to practice self-forgiveness. In fact, when they are unsuccessful, it is more likely for the perfectionist to be especially hard on themselves.

I have also observed interesting correlations between perfectionism and various health ailments and disorders. An example of this is the connection between clients with multiple sclerosis and high expectations. Perfectionism seems to be a strong component in almost every MS client with whom I have worked. It is as if the internal attack that is occurring within the body of a multiple sclerosis patient mirrors the self-criticism that someone with high expectations will inflict upon themselves. The result of this appears to be a body so overwhelmed by the fear of failure and the need to control that it manifests a disease where the individual experiences a *loss of control*. This is something I have seen in my practice, but to my knowledge there are no scientific studies or evidence that corroborates this observation.

ACTIVITY FOR LOVING YOURSELF

The objective of this activity is to provide an opportunity for you to participate in a task without having the need to win or control or excel or perform perfectly for yourself or anyone in your life. The goal is to throw out all pressure to perform and take part in something where the only stipulation is to love yourself unconditionally throughout the process. No criticism is allowed.

Step 1
Gather a few art supplies such as a paintbrush, paints (watercolors, poster, or acrylic paints), and a large piece of paper, which will be your canvas.

Step 2
Set aside ninety minutes where you know you will not be disturbed.

Step 3
Set the timer for ninety minutes. You have ninety minutes to complete your painting. It does not have to be a picture of something—it can be a freestyle expression of color and shapes. Since quality is *not* important, the goal is to use as many colors as possible (no, the brush doesn't need to be thoroughly cleaned each time you change colors), cover every inch of the paper, and the painting *must* be finished within the ninety minute time frame. Completing only a small part of the painting or wanting to come back and spend a couple more hours at a later time implies that something about your painting is not good enough. That is not allowed. The objective is for you to love it and to love yourself during every minute of this process. Absolutely no criticism or negative

self-talk is allowed during any part of this activity. If you start to feel like a kid again as you do this, that is wonderful. Allow yourself to connect with those feelings because there might be a part of you that was never allowed this degree of freedom and fun as a child.

Do it for the pure joy of having fun and feeling free.

Step 4

Take a minute and laugh at yourself, at this process, and perhaps at your painting. The objective is to have fun. No one has to see this except you. Since this is a spontaneous work from your heart, when you are finished you are only allowed to admire it and say nice things about the finished product.

In Their Own Words

Helen and her husband were in a situation where they had to rely on medical technology and use an in vitro procedure in order to get pregnant. Helen turned to hypnosis because she was experiencing a very high level of stress associated with the medical procedures and trying to get pregnant.

It was easier for Helen to be objective and understand her perfectionist tendencies because two of the activities Helen took part in when she was younger, ballet and ice skating, were activities that demanded perfection. After identifying the source of the internal pressure, Helen was able to use techniques such as meditation and visualization to reduce her anxiety and get her body to move out of the stress response or fight-or-flight mode. In doing this work, Helen was able to bring her body and emotions back to a healthy balanced state where conception was possible.

Helen's Story
The Emotional Journey

When I first found out that my husband and I would have to go through IVF to get pregnant I was extremely upset, concerned, worried, and scared. However, we wanted a baby so badly that we were willing to do anything to reach our dream and have our family. Due to the cost of IVF, we decided to participate in a study that would pay for the majority of the process. However, getting started was quite a challenge. On the first day, when I went in to start the IVF medications, they did the ultrasound to make sure my ovaries were good, and told me to come back later that day. We were so excited, but then we received a phone call that I did not weigh enough to be in the study and needed to gain about fifteen pounds. Over the next month I stuffed myself and did everything possible to gain the weight. The following month I weighed in at 132 pounds, so I was ready to start. But then when they checked my ovaries, they found a cyst and once again I was told I could not start the process. I was so frustrated and upset, and thought I'd never get to start, but finally, after waiting another month, we went back for the third time, and I had no cysts and weighed enough so we could start the IVF medication. My husband and I both cried because we were finally on our way to starting a family.

It was quite an emotional roller-coaster, going through all the hormone injections and growing the eggs, but we made it through and they were able to fertilize enough eggs. The day they called me in for the transfer, I was so excited. They transferred two embryos and then I had to be on bed rest for a few days. I was so anxious and worried during those next two weeks while I waited to find out if I was pregnant. I was very emotional and stressed and kept wondering if I was pregnant or not. On Mother's Day, I went in to do a pregnancy test. I was so scared and nervous and excited, but later that afternoon the nurse called with the most devastating call I had ever received. I was not pregnant. I had never cried so much in my life and never felt so hopeless. After all we had gone through just to get to this point, and it had failed.

The next day we talked to the doctor, who had no explanation for why it did not work, but he was very hopeful that I would get pregnant and wanted us to try again with the frozen embryos. So we decided to try again right away, but this time I added acupuncture and hypnotherapy to help. I started doing acupuncture once a week, which helped relax and calm me. I also went to hypnotherapy once a week, which allowed me to get in touch with myself and look at some underlying subconscious issues that I needed to deal with.

Undergoing the hypnosis and learning meditation techniques helped me immensely. The meditation helped me to relax and calm my nerves while I was going through the IVF process for the second time, and it helped me feel in tune with my body. Through hypnosis I was able to clear some emotional blocks that I had. One of the largest was my perfectionism. For many years I was a competitive ice skater and ballet dancer, both sports which require perfection. I trained for years by perfecting the moves and landing jumps to win competitions, and I was hard on myself when I made mistakes. Even in school, I wanted to do everything perfect and always get straight A's. Amazingly I never got a B in my life, and graduated valedictorian from high school, summa cum laude in college and with high honors in my master's degree program. But in dealing with IVF and pregnancy, I had no control, and even if I followed all the rules and did everything right, there were no guarantees. Hypnosis helped me to work through these feelings and realize that it was okay and I wasn't a failure. In addition, it helped to release any emotional baggage from my past and let go of any pain, anger, and stress that might be preventing fertility.

Through the meditation and visualization techniques, I was able to get in touch with my body, relax my internal self and visualize the embryos implanting. I practiced this every day for a month before the next embryo transfer, so that on the day of the transfer I was ready. The difference in how I felt this second time was incredible. Yes, I was still a little nervous and anxious, but this time I felt positive and calm and ready. During the procedure I went into a meditative state, and it was honestly the deepest meditation/hypnosis that I have been in. I felt my body completely relaxed and

energy running through me… it was incredible. During my period of bed rest, I stayed with my parents, and even my parents
noticed the dramatic difference in my stress level this time. My
husband was impressed with how calm and relaxed I seemed.
Through the next week I continued meditating and talking with
the embryos.

Then finally, it was the day of the pregnancy test. It was hard
to remain calm since the replay of the nurse's disappointing
phone call was still in my head. But I went in thinking positively,
because deep down, internally, I felt I was pregnant. We waited
all day for the phone call, and I started getting very nervous and
anxious, when finally the phone rang. My husband answered because I was too anxious, but the nurse would not tell him, so he
passed me the phone. My heart stopped, and then I heard, "I
wanted to be the first to congratulate you…. YOU'RE PREG-
NANT!" I just started screaming and crying and experienced every
emotion possible. Joy and excitement overcame me. We did
it…. all the hard work and waiting, and I was finally pregnant!

I truly believe that the hypnotherapy and acupuncture had a
huge role in our success. It helped lower my stress level, help me
feel positive, and prepared me mentally and spiritually. I am in
no way discounting the medical aspect of IVF, because without
the experienced doctors this would have never been possible, but
I do believe that the mind-body/hypnosis work was just as important to the process.

CHAPTER EIGHT

REPROGRAMMING AT THE CELLULAR LEVEL

This chapter is about how the cells in our bodies listen and respond to our thoughts, beliefs, attitudes, and environment. Some readers have scientific minds and want research and technical information, while others simply want to know how the latest cellular discoveries relate to their ability to conceive. There are a few moments in this chapter where it gets a little technical; however, the general concepts presented here are very important because scientific evidence now supports the fact that our thought patterns can have a profound influence on whether or not the cells and the body support or resist conception. This means that we may have more control over the ability to get pregnant than we ever imagined. It also opens up the possibility of mind-body healing, at the cellular level, which offers great hope and potential to enhance the fertility process.

OUR CELLS ARE LISTENING

New discoveries in science are unfolding so rapidly that it seems like the textbooks, and many of our old assumptions about biology, have quickly become outdated. One of those old beliefs—which has been proven false—is the assumption that our cells have rigid programming and simply carry out their specific functions while being oblivious to the outside world. Biologists now know that cells are *not* impartial microscopic forms with rigid programming; instead, our cells are continually changing, responding, and reacting to stimuli from their environment.

The term "environment," also referred to as the *field*, is what might be described as the big picture. The field encompasses everything from our living environment—such as the air we breathe, the water we drink, and the influence of the people around us—to our own private world. Our private world includes such things as what we eat, how we experience physical activity, how we feel about ourselves, how much stress and anxiety we feel and so on. In other words, the field or environment means everything in our existence: thoughts, beliefs, and feelings; how we nurture and care for our physical bodies; and the world we live in, whether that be a peaceful house in the country or the excitement and chaos of a big city.

When the environment sends information to our cells, it is received by a part of the cell membrane called the cell receptors (see figure 8.1). According to Anne Trafton, describing the recent discoveries at the Massachusetts Institute of Technology, "Receptors on the cell surface allow the cell to maintain constant communication with its environment— they bind to molecules that convey information about the environment and instructions telling them what functions to carry out."[1] Cell receptors are sensors that receive the signal or message from the field and communicate that information to the cell, and then the cell responds accordingly. Our cells are *not* insensitive to signals from the environment—on the contrary—they are constantly absorbing, responding, and reacting to stimuli. Our cells are listening to every message we convey.

For each message a cell receives, it creates a corresponding response. For example, the cells within the body of someone who exists in a stressful environment might receive an anxiety signal and respond by producing cortisol, increasing the heart rate, constricting blood vessels, or creating a skin rash, depending on where those cells are located in the body. The reaction may start with the brain cells, or neurons, which can sense the stressful situation and then convey that information via chemical message carriers, known as neuropeptides, to the appropriate cells and organs that carry out the physical manifestations of the stress response. *Our cells are listening and reacting to every impulse in our environment.* As Dr. Deepak Chopra, an advocate of mind-body healing, says in *Magical Mind, Magical Body*, "We have a thinking body…. The mind is

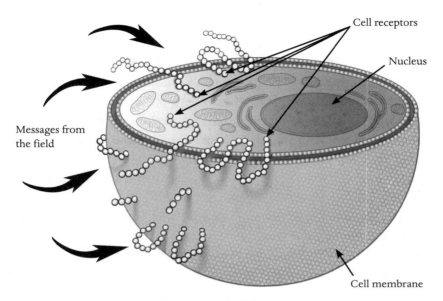

Cell receptors

Nucleus

Messages from
the field

Cell membrane

Figure 8.1: Cell receptors and cellular communication.

not confined to the brain. The mind is in every cell of the body."[2] In the
past, the body was viewed as simply a physical structure having the ability to carry out chemical and biological functions. It was thought of in
scientific terms with no connection to thought or perception. That is
no longer true. It is now known that the cells of the body are listening,
thinking, and responding to every signal they receive.

Since our cells are continually responding to the information they
receive, then it is important to look at the messages that are being sent.
A good message might create a positive response in the body as in the
case where a relaxing massage might increase the production of endorphins, those peptides that make us feel relaxed and happy.

What happens when a negative impulse is sent to the cells? For example, how do the cells respond when a woman is told by her doctor that
she may never have children naturally because she is too old? The initial
reaction within her body, when she hears those words, would likely be
one of intense feelings of sadness and grief. The consequence of the
grieving might be a message to her body that she has abandoned all hope
of a natural pregnancy and is giving up on her dream. That information

may generate instructions to her cells, telling them that they no longer need to expend energy in trying to support conception. What happens when the follicles, the ovaries, the uterus, the hypothalamus gland, and the gland responsible for hormones—the pituitary—receive this message? If this is the information the cells receive from the environment, it seems likely that they will follow those orders. Remember, the physical body is not simply a scientific machine: the body is thinking, sensing, and responding to everything around us.

What about the woman who feels overwhelmed by stress—from her infertility and from life in general? Could that anxiety work its way to the cells of the hypothalamus and pituitary glands—the brain's control centers for reproduction—and interrupt the proper balance of hormones to promote conception? Could her hypothalamus gland interpret that stressful signal as a sign that this woman is feeling fearful and vulnerable and therefore her body should not be reproducing? The scientific evidence has proven that the hypothalamus *does* respond adversely to stress. This is yet another example of how the mind-body connection is reacting to its environment.

What about a woman who, when she was younger, spent much of her life being scared to death about having an unwanted pregnancy. Perhaps she had a couple of relationships with partners whom she knew weren't right for her, and spent the better part of two decades telling her reproductive system, "No matter what, don't let me get pregnant." The cells in her uterus might have interpreted that signal as: "Don't allow anything to implant. If any object tries to grow within the uterus, it should be expelled." Then, as things changed in her life and she found a wonderful partner, she decides she wants to get pregnant through an IVF procedure. What is the long-term programming within her uterine cells? Are those cells still following the orders of the past about preventing pregnancy at all costs, and could that affect the efficacy of the in vitro implantation? It seems like her chances of success could be greatly enhanced if a new message could rewrite the information that her cells received in the past. Our cells are listening now, but they have also been listening in the past.

The information within our cells, and the external programming that continually communicates to our cell receptors, can have a profound influence on our physiology. I believe that there are ways to change or heal old information by reprogramming the information and belief systems embedded in our cells.

OUR CELLS ARE CHANGING

We are continually replacing the old cells in our bodies with new ones. That is a biological fact. Some cells are replaced in a matter of days, others take months. It is almost as if we are rebuilding our entire bodies—a cell at a time—every three to twelve months. Dr. Deepak Chopra says:

> You replace 98 percent of all of the atoms in your body in less than one year. You make a new liver every six months, a new skeleton once every three months, a new stomach lining every five days and a new skin once a month. Even the brain cells that you think with as physical atoms, they weren't there last year.[3]

Therefore, the notion of healing or reprogramming our cells opens up intriguing possibilities, especially if the new cells that are created could be generated with a new consciousness or belief system. And what if the new cells were programmed for healing and we could replace the old unhealthy cells with healthy new ones? This opens up tremendous opportunities for mind-body healing.

While scientists agree that our bodies are continually generating new cells, in the past they have also believed that some of the most important cells necessary to make this process possible—neurons—are fixed at birth (see figure 8.2). Neurons are cells that are present in our brains and nervous systems, and they are some of our most important cells because these cells influence how we think and feel. If these cells are fixed at birth and can't accept new ideas or beliefs and can't be regenerated, it would suggest that we could be limited in integrating new programming that might positively affect our lives. New science has now proven that those old beliefs about fixed, unchangeable neurons to be untrue. Neurons *are* being regenerated and they *are* very responsive to signals from their environment.

Scientist have now witnessed a process called neurogenesis in which new neurons grow and develop in the brain. Research led by Peter Eriksson of Sweden and Fred Gage of the Salk Institute found that "neurogenesis occurs in the brains of adult humans as old as seventy-two years of age! This neurogenesis is believed to be due to neural stem cells that exist in the adult human brain."[4] Due to the fact that neurons are so complex and specialized, researchers had assumed that it wouldn't be possible for new neurons to grow and develop. The neurogenesis research showed that new neurons could be generated from stem cells. Stem cells are present throughout our bodies, and it is believed that stem cells may be very active in the process of cell generation. *This opens the door, not only for future scientific work, but also for the possibilities in mind-body healing.* If the most complex cells in our bodies can be regenerated, and we already know that simpler cells undergo this process, this creates exciting possibilities for healing work. It suggests that we could bring in new cells with a different belief system or replace unhealthy cells with vital cells programmed for positive change. For example, could stem cells be used to rejuvenate and then stimulate the release of healthier follicles? Could they be used to replace cells where endometriosis is present in the reproductive system? And how much of this could be done with mind-body techniques?

Naturally, for mind-body healing to take place, the neurons in our brains must be able to respond. If neurons are fixed and unchangeable, it would mean that a new belief could never replace an old one. In actuality, neurons provide some of the best evidence that our cells are responding and listening to information from the environment. Neurons carry messages or nerve impulses. The interconnections between neurons (see figure 8.2) are called synapses; when the connection between neurons, made via those synapses, changes, it is called plasticity. This phenomenon has been proven in recent studies conducted at Brown University where researchers observed neurons responding to stimuli as "the brain's ability to reorganize itself—strengthening or weakening connections between neurons or adding or subtracting those connections..."⁵ Changes in the neurons and synaptic connections indicate that new thoughts are *continually* being integrated into our belief system and transmitted to our bodies. Our cells and bodies are cognizant and changeable. We can take an idea such as "My FSH is too high to get pregnant naturally" and change it to "Through mind-body healing and acupuncture, I am creating healthy, perfect follicles." Will that work? Is there scientific proof? The studies in chapter two indicate that working with the mind seems to have a profound influence on one's ability to get pregnant. Those studies indicate that it is time to approach the promotion of conception from a new perspective. While those studies may have approached the situation by addressing the whole person, the information in this chapter shows that there is evidence, at a *cellular level*, that we are listening, responding, and making changes within our bodies based on the information we absorb from our field.

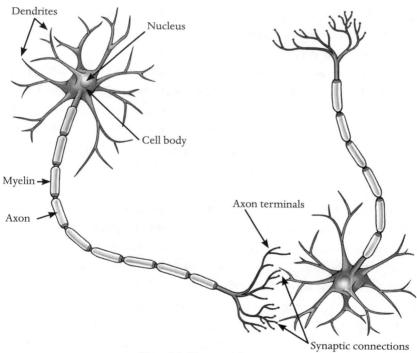

Figure 8.2: Neurons and synapses.

What does all this scientific information mean to someone who is trying to get pregnant? We are not fixed and unchangeable. Our thoughts, beliefs, and attitudes can have a profound influence on the ability to have a baby. Scientific evidence demonstrates that our cells are constantly receiving and responding to stimuli. It suggests that our cells are not static and they *do* react to the environment. It opens the potential for healing and reprogramming some of the physical issues that might be interfering with conception. Since we know our cells are listening and changing, the question becomes: what messages are we sending?

THE DNA FACTOR

Some might respond by saying, "okay, my cells are listening but my problem is in my genes. It runs in my family, and it is part of my genetic make-up." This could be women who say things like: "All the women in my family have trouble getting pregnant." "All the women in my family have cycles that are too short." "My follicles are not viable; it must be something in my genes."

Old beliefs about our genes and the information in our DNA, the strands of proteins that contain our genetic material, have also been modified to reflect new discoveries in recent years. In the past, DNA has been regarded as *fixed* programming that never changed. Whatever traits were in your genes were programmed into your DNA and subsequently would manifest in the physical body. Dr. Bruce Lipton, a cell biologist and former professor and researcher at Stanford University, is one of a number of scientists who are changing our understanding of cellular functions. Perhaps the most significant awakening has come in our understanding of DNA. Lipton, in his book *The Biology of Belief*, explains how new discoveries have changed the way we see the role of DNA and the impact of the field on the actions of a cell: "... a cell's life is controlled by the physical and energetic environment and *not* by its genes.... It is a single cell's 'awareness' of the environment, not its genes, that sets into motion the mechanisms of life."[6] Lipton goes on to say that not only is the cell itself responding and changing based on the environment, but so is the DNA within our cells and that cells have the ability *to activate or not activate* the programming within the DNA based on the information they receive:

> ... DNA blueprints passed down through genes are not set in concrete at birth. Genes are not destiny! Environmental influences, including nutrition, stress, and emotions, can modify those genes, without changing their basic blueprint.[7]

This means that the information from the field is responsible for the messages sent to the DNA of each cell, and it is that information that brings about cellular reactions or mechanisms by which genes can either be set into motion or the body and cells can choose not to activate a gene and instead create a different physiological response. These new discoveries are incredibly significant because they challenge our traditional beliefs about the functions and fixed programming of DNA. It implies that our DNA responds to our actions and beliefs and is *not* predestined to follow a fixed set of behaviors and instructions.

If DNA is not set in stone, that means that genetic profiling or genetic determinism, the practice of predicting what traits—positive or negative—will occur in our bodies, loses much of its validity. For example, Craig Venter, a member of one of the teams who cracked the human genome, says that having the colon cancer gene in one's DNA does *not* necessarily mean an individual will develop colon cancer. "Even though some patients carry this mutated gene in every cell, the cancer only occurs in the colon because it is triggered by toxins secreted by bacteria in the gut. Cancer, argues Venter, is an environmental disease ..." The environment is a huge player in whether or not that cancer will actually occur.[8]

More and more experts who have worked on unraveling the human genome have come out against the idea that our biology is rigidly controlled by DNA, and they are now asserting that environment plays a crucial role. Genetic specialist Dr. Kevin Davies states, "The seesaw struggle between our genes (nature) and the environment (nurture) [has] swung sharply in favor of nurture,"[9] meaning that old belief of "it's in my genes," is no longer valid. Our health is now directly determined by thoughts, beliefs, levels of stress, diet, environmental contaminants, and a number of other factors that make up the field.

A landmark study which looked at the effects of genes vs. environment on twins recently took place in Sweden. At issue was that if twins have similar DNA, then if a disharmony occurs in the body of one twin, it should occur in the other. Researchers found that assumption to be completely false, which indicates that our DNA is *not* controlling what happens in our bodies. It was a huge blow to the old beliefs that all of the outcomes of our health were determined by DNA. It made it clear that just because someone carries a cancer gene in their DNA, it does not mean that cancer will ever become a reality. The conclusion of that study made a powerful statement about preexisting views regarding genetic determinism. It specifically addressed the old misconceptions about how having a gene that is a marker for cancer meant that the disease was a certainty:

> The relative roles of genes and environment in the development of cancer have been debated for years. It is now generally accepted that only 10–20 percent of all cancers are genetically "preordained" while the remaining 80–90 percent are caused by wrong diet, infections, or by excessive exposure to carcinogens such as tobacco, alcohol, radiation, occupational toxins, and drugs.[10]

This study, which looked at 44,788 pairs of twins, was so extensive that critics who often try to debunk studies for being too small had no grounds on which to base objections. While the researchers said that some cancers have a larger genetic component than others, they "confirmed that the overall contribution of genetic constitution to the risk of all cancers is about 15 percent."[11]

The conclusion of the study was especially significant. It clearly states that doctors and geneticists cannot determine an individual's risk of cancer based on their genes:

The researchers concluded that the heritable component of cancer is not a very significant risk factor even among close relatives. Dr. Robert Hoover, MD, of the National Cancer Institute lauds the new study and points out that it clearly shows the futility of trying to predict an individual's risk of cancer from their genetic constitution.[12]

This statement, coming from a doctor who represents the National Cancer Institute, sends a deliberate message about the shortcomings of genetic predestination.

What this means about genetic determinism is that "... we are not victims of our genes, but masters of our fates ..."[13] It is time to let go of the fatalistic thinking and old beliefs about cells being preprogrammed and understand that our cells are constantly responding to signals coming from our thoughts and the world around us. A gene within our DNA *does not* mean that this is our predetermined fate. Genetic testing can be very misleading because genetic issues *do not* have to be expressed or set in motion. Again, the key is the signal, the thought, and the lifestyle—for each individual that is different. With this knowledge, we can take responsibility for our health.

What do these discoveries mean for infertility? Any thoughts that a woman's situation might be the result of heredity may be more about her belief system than what is in her genes. Any fixed beliefs or negative messages being communicated to the cells may need to be reevaluated. Any physical conditions that might be blocking conception may be something that can be addressed with mind-body work and/or alternative modalities. It creates new hope and attacks old beliefs that can make us feel trapped and like victims of our genetic make-up.

THE ORIGINS OF THE MESSAGES
WE SEND TO OUR CELLS

One of the essential elements in making these changes is to identify the source or origins of the messages and programming that is being communicated to our cells. The most powerful information that shapes who we are is coming from the subconscious mind. One's conscious mind might be saying all the right things and sending positive signals, but the subconscious mind (see chapter three for more information about the conscious and subconscious minds) is far more powerful. It doesn't do any good to repeat a daily affirmation saying, "I will get pregnant," if there are overriding subconscious beliefs counteracting those positive thoughts with feelings like: "I'm not sure if I can be a good mother," or "I don't deserve to get pregnant because of some of the things I've done in my past," or "My FSH is too high for me to get pregnant." *The material in the subconscious mind is far more powerful than any form of conscious thought.* If the subconscious mind is sending old negative beliefs, that information can easily override the messages from the conscious mind.

Dr. Deepak Chopra says that the average person "thinks 60,000 thoughts a day. Ninety-five percent of those are the same thoughts we had yesterday, creating the same patterns that give rise to the same physical expression of the body."[14] In other words, we are continually reinforcing the same old beliefs. Those same beliefs can keep us stuck in an infertility mindset and a physical body receiving continual messages about how it is failing to perform. In order for us to change our physiology, we have to change the way we think, because that changes the messages or *instructions* that are sent to the cells.

GENETIC DETERMINISM
AND THE SUBCONSCIOUS MIND

The belief in genetic determinism presents a particularly dangerous dilemma because once a powerful idea is introduced to the subconscious, it can easily become part of one's belief system, and in turn send those signals to the cells in our bodies. For example, if they isolated a gene that governed ovarian reserve and a woman had a marker that indicated she would always have poor follicle quality, what would prevent her from allowing this to become her reality. Thoughts are incredibly powerful, and receiving news like that could build a huge wall between that woman and a successful pregnancy.

The same might be true when a doctor tells a woman she has the breast cancer gene. She might start believing that diagnosis and begin sending that information—through her thoughts and fears—to her cells. In a sense, she might be creating the disease. I believe that it is possible that knowledge of a genetic marker in the hands of some people might create the fearful cellular programming that, in turn, makes the body create that illness. We may have a better answer to that question in the next few years as more studies in genetic testing and subsequent behavioral outcomes come to light.

HOW WE CAN USE THIS NEW SCIENCE TO OUR ADVANTAGE

While key components of environment include things such as the food we put in our bodies and elements, like toxins, in our physical world, I believe that *thought* is one of the most important elements of our environment. It is important to hold a clear vision of what we want to create as our reality. Our thoughts manifest into what we see occurring in our lives. There are many ways this plays out, and the evidence here indicates that it is occurring even at the cellular level. If a woman spends 90 percent of her day worrying that she will never get pregnant, what is her energy manifesting or creating in her body? What signal is she sending to her cells? Is it fear and lack or is it fertility and vibrant health? On the other hand, the woman who visualizes the conception process happening inside of her, every day, is also shaping her destiny. Our thoughts become what we create in our lives.

The field or environment is us co-creating our future. If a woman learns that she has high FSH and as a result makes sweeping changes in her life—a healthy diet, cuts out the overtime at her job, resolves old issues, learns to meditate, and adopts the belief that she is fertile—there is a good chance she will positively affect what is happening in her body. Conversely, the woman who gets the same diagnosis but changes nothing in her field or environment is unlikely to see any improvement in this area.

The environment includes not only our thoughts and beliefs, but also the input of the people around us. If a woman experiencing infertility is in a family with a fatalistic attitude about her chances, that energy and negativity may also be sending a message to her cells. Continual sentiments like, "you can always adopt" imply that she is never going to be successful. Success is more likely to be achieved while being surrounded with positive supporting friends who resonate with the idea of seeing new possibilities.

This is why the ideal fertility support group could best be described as one that is positive and healing. Granted, there are times when negative emotions may need to be discussed in a group, but if the focus is on healing, then the cells receive a message that they are healing. I have clients who attend infertility support groups and report back that every time they return from a meeting, they come home feeling drained and depressed and hopeless. Those aren't the signals we want our cells to receive.

This doesn't mean that we go into denial about our situations. It is impossible to stay positive all of the time. A suitable compromise might be to send positive messages to the cells 90 percent of the time with the understanding that there will be some negative feelings that creep in the other 10 percent of the time. It isn't realistic to believe that we could eliminate negative thoughts completely.

The most positive news, from the biological standpoint, is the stem cells that I mentioned earlier in this chapter. The belief about stem cells is that their purpose is to help us regenerate new healthy cells to replace the old. The possibilities with stem cells appear to be almost limitless. The current perception is that there are millions of stem cells in our bodies waiting for signals to call them to action. There are numerous possibilities for scientific and mind-body healing in this area, and someone who believes that this is possible sends a clear signal to their cells in regard to what they want to achieve. Some methods of working with stem cells include the practices of acupuncture and mind-body healing programs such as meditation and hypnosis. I believe the most effective method to work with mind-body cellular reprogramming is hypnosis.

In deep meditation and hypnosis it is easy to access the theta state (a brain-wave state characterized by deep relaxation) which is more receptive to new information and healing. So, if a woman wants to potentiate the work she is doing, those two modalities can help make her work more powerful. In the psychotherapeutic field, it is not acceptable to say "cellular healing," because that implies it is a medical process. The term one might see associated with cell work is likely to be something like cellular reprogramming.

Is there an iron-clad guarantee that these modalities are scientifically proven and will work? No. But we all have choices in regard to our healing. We can take responsibility for our healing or decide to become victims and let fate take over, but remember, either way, we are sending a message to our cells.

Can this create false hope as some critics might say? I don't believe so. I don't think we've tapped into even a small percentage of what the mind can do. My belief is that when you attempt something, such as getting pregnant, it feels better to know that one is doing everything possible to create success. Women often tell me that they'd rather look back at this time in their life and say, "I tried everything," instead of, "I wish I had done more."

So, what is the vision *you* are sending to your cells? What do you want to create in your life? The exercise below is an important start in shaping your future. Instead of coming from a place of fear and doubt, this exercise will help you change the signals that you send your cells. The more this message—or meditation—is repeated, the more it becomes part of the belief system of your subconscious mind.

EXERCISE: VISUALIZING YOUR FUTURE

Make a list of all the negative thoughts you have about getting pregnant. This could be things like: I have a low ovarian reserve. My doctor says I have only a 2 percent chance of getting pregnant because of my age. I'm worried that I may not be a good mother.

Now take that list and rewrite the information that you've been sending to your cells. Make all of the messages positive and write them in present tense. For example, the list above might change to this: I am young and healthy. I am taking good care of my body and producing perfect, healthy follicles. I am a gentle, loving person and a great mother.

Close your eyes, take ten deep breaths, and enter a meditative state. Repeat each of the positive statements that you've written above. To make them more powerful, imagine yourself in scenes where you visualize yourself manifesting what each statement is saying. For example, as you say, "I am a gentle, loving person and a great mother," imagine yourself in a scene where you are playing and having a great time with your children.

It may feel a little awkward at first. That is your subconscious trying to run some interference with thoughts like "that will never happen" or "I'm going to make you struggle to imagine something that wonderful." It is yet another indication that the subconscious material is present in all of us. Those resisting thoughts should go away as you process your issues. You might consider making a recording of these statements so that you can listen to them every day. That way, you are repeatedly sending positive messages to your cells to replace the old programming.

In Their Own Words

This story is a testament to how our thoughts, attitudes, and beliefs—a key component of the field—can influence our physiology.

Elizabeth mentions that before she started doing mind-body work, she would walk into each procedure believing, "It isn't going to work either." That information was being communicated to and providing the programming of her cells.

Elizabeth felt that her parents would be disappointed if she had children. Since the field encompasses the environment around us, including our families, this belief can create yet another obstacle to interfere with conception. It is natural for children—even children who have grown into adults—to want to please their parents. The message Elizabeth's body received from this was that if she became pregnant, she would be letting her parents down.

Elizabeth reduced her stress and changed the information that she sent to her cells. Not only did this work for her IVF procedure, but she also overcame the "eggs were too old" programming—yet another message from the field—and was able to conceive naturally.

Elizabeth's Story
Working With Meditation

Before starting with hypnosis, we had gone through four years of trying naturally. We had done fertility tests and were told that we had unexplained infertility, although they did say that my eggs were too old and that was the issue. The doctor always said I would never be able to get pregnant naturally, and even if I did, I wouldn't be able to carry to term because my eggs were no good. We'd gone though several fertility treatments including clomid, IUI, and I had tried an IVF with my own eggs that failed. Then, I did a transfer with donor eggs that failed, despite the fact that everything looked wonderful. We were definitely at the last straw when we started hypnosis.

We were under so much stress with everything we had done and all the bad news we had been getting that the hypnotherapy really helped put a positive focus on our situation. It helped us adopt a positive attitude, and positive energy rather than walking in with the assumption that "the next procedure isn't going to work either." It really helped deal with the stress, to be able to relax and put things into perspective and believe that, one way or another, things were going to come out okay. If I could turn the hands of time back, early in this process, I would have started this sooner and avoided all this stress.

There were some emotional blocks that I had to work through in the hypnosis sessions. I specifically remember feeling an expected reaction of disappointment from my parents when I made the phone call to say I was having a child. I expected—instead of excitement—a simple response of "Oh." I was raised to believe that career was most important and family just slows you down. In one session, I distinctly remembered, at a young age, having a conversation with my mom where this was reinforced. I was able to acknowledge that for what it was and move beyond it.

Working with meditation helped with the stress as well as shifting my entire thought pattern. Building on what we did in our sessions, I'd go back in my own meditations, and reinforce everything positively, believing everything was going to turn out okay, rather than letting all my negative thoughts creep in and end up walking into another doctor's appointment expecting failure and bad news. I still use the meditation today to deal with everything else that goes on, and I definitely feel I am a much happier and healthier person for it.

I believe that hypnosis played a big part in being able to get pregnant with my son through IVF. A lot of this almost seemed like magic to me. I was also doing acupuncture, and seeing a naturopathic doctor and feel like all of those things helped me a great deal.

After the work we did together, not only was I able to have a successful pregnancy with a donor egg, but two years later, even though I'd never been pregnant naturally before, I did get pregnant on my own, two times in a row after the first birth. Unfortunately, I lost the first one, but now I have a very happy, healthy ten-month-old—and that was a completely natural pregnancy. Anybody I talk to who is going through infertility, I recommend hypnosis and acupuncture. I believe those modalities got us to the success of having the family we were looking for as well as improving my physical and mental well-being, probably for the rest of my life.

WORKS CITED

1. Trafton, Anne, "Force, not light, gives researchers images of cell receptors." http://web.mit.edu/newsoffice/2007/cell-receptor-0613.html, June 13, 2007.

2. Deepak, Chopra, *Magical Mind, Magical Body: Mastering the Mind-body Connection for Perfect Health and Total Well-Being.* Audio CD (Nightingale Conant, 1991), CD # 1, Track 3.

3. Ibid. CD # 1, Track 2.

4. John Pinel, "Neurogenesis in the Adult Human Brain." From the Biopsychology site, http://www.abacon.com/pinel/hot_sept.html.

5. Wendy Lawton, "What Can Change the Brain? Electrical Synapses, Research Shows." Press Release from Brown University, http://www.brown.edu/Administration/News_Bureau/2005–06/05–055.html, December 15, 2005.

6. Bruce Lipton, *The Biology of Belief* (Santa Rosa, CA: Mountain of Love/Elite Books, 2005), 15.

7. Ibid., 67.

8. Kevin, Davies, "Nature vs. Nurture Revisited." From Nova Online, http://www.pbs.org/wgbh/nova/genome/debate.html.

9. Ibid.

10. Paul Lichtenstein, et al, "Environmental and heritable factors in the causation of cancer: analyses of cohorts of twins from Sweden, Denmark, and Finland," *New England Journal of Medicine*, Vol. 343 (July 13, 2000): pp. 78–85.

11. Ibid., pp. 78–85.

12. Lichtenstein, et al, "Environmental and heritable factors." Hoover, Robert N. "Cancer—Nature, nurture, or both," *New England Journal of Medicine*, Vol. 343 (July 13, 2000): pp. 135–36 (editorial).

13. Lipton, "The Biology of Belief," 27.

14. Chopra, "Magical Mind," CD # 1, Track 4.

CHAPTER NINE

WORKING WITH MEDITATION
AND VISUALIZATION

Meditation is a healing process. It has been well documented that meditation is not only beneficial for decreasing stress, but it also affects our physical health in a positive way by doing such things as lowering the heart rate and, if it tends to run high, reducing blood pressure. By spending a few minutes each day in meditation, people become more grounded and focused and consequently become more efficient in their jobs. A calm mind can function at a higher level and is better equipped to perform under pressure. In short, meditation provides health benefits, reduces stress, increases our sense of well-being, makes us more productive, and can open the door to mind-body healing.

So, why are people who practice meditation every day in the minority? Part of the reason may be that it was never a part of Western culture. Although it is practiced in many other cultures around the world, many of us were never exposed to meditation. Some, who branched out and wanted to learn what meditation was all about, learned practices that may have taught them to empty their head and think of nothing, which can be beneficial, but is nearly impossible for the majority of us to do. Most people simply never had direction and guidance in this area, and it is a practice that is often difficult to learn on our own. It is one of those disciplines where it helps to have someone to guide or teach the process so that the technique can be customized to meet our individual needs.

Meditation is an essential part of the fertility journey. It not only aids in letting go of stress and tension, but it provides the opportunity to incorporate mind-body healing and process the issues that may be getting in the way of conception. I have all of my clients work with meditation because this daily process is like having a ten-minute reinforcement session every day. Old subconscious material is so deeply ingrained that it requires more than the once-a-week sessions to make lasting changes. The old beliefs and programming have been reinforced for years or, in many cases, decades. Changing that programming requires new input *on a daily basis* until the existing information gives way to the new. The work done in an actual hypnosis session—uncovering and processing old beliefs and emotions that block our success—is absolutely vital to making positive changes, but the daily follow-up work is crucial to the process of creating a new subconscious paradigm. The only way to do that work—when not in the presence of a practitioner— is as a daily process in a meditative state, and it is this follow-up work that creates permanent changes in our lives.

After completing a hypnosis session, most clients feel like they have a positive attitude, feel confident about themselves, and believe they will be successful. However, with the stresses of daily life, it is easy to find ourselves bounced right back to where we started, experiencing old doubts and fears. Meditation can help us recapture the mindset and attitude we experienced during the session. It can help us regain focus on the goals that are important to us and return to a relaxed state.

Because we all have our own unique stuff to reprogram, it is best to have a meditation that is designed to meet our personal needs. There are meditation-for-fertility CDs which can be great for general relaxation and visualizing conception, but I believe it is most beneficial to engage in a personalized daily meditation that specifically addresses the areas of need for the *individual*. For example, one client may be working on mind-body healing for high FSH, processing a miscarriage, and releasing perfectionism, while another client might be lowering stress, forgiving and releasing abuse and dysfunction in her birth family, and building her self-concept. These two women require very different meditative processes, and it is not possible for these things to be addressed in a CD that is available for sale to the general public. So, the purchase of generalized CDs is quite beneficial for stress reduction and generalized visualization, but to maximize success and create lasting changes at the subconscious level, it is most advantageous to have a meditation formulated by a practitioner that addresses the needs and goals of the individual.

SCIENTIFIC EVIDENCE

While there have been many studies touting the benefits of meditation, one of the most significant was a landmark study performed at Harvard Medical School under the direction of Dr. Herbert Benson in 1967. Benson, a cardiologist and Associate Professor of Medicine at Harvard, wasn't sure how the scientific community would respond to a study which measured the effects of meditation on our physiology, so he would sneak a group of thirty-six transcendental meditators into his lab late at night in order to monitor their progress. He found that people in meditation "used 17 percent less oxygen, lowered their heart rate by three beats a minute and increased their theta brain waves..."[1] Benson published his work in a book called *The Relaxation Response*. It showed how "ten minutes of meditative technique a day could increase concentration and counteract the harmful effects of stress, such as high blood pressure and strokes."[2]

When talking about the benefits of mind-body processes, it seems like there are always skeptics who express their doubts, so it is interesting to note that one company in an industry that typically does not support alternative modalities is now encouraging the use of meditation and visualization. Blue Shield of California, one of the major health insurance companies, has instituted a guided imagery program that includes distributing meditation CDs to patients who are preparing for surgery. Why would a major insurance company embrace a practice that has at times been dismissed by the scientific community? The reason is because it is successful, and it is saving the company money. Blue Shield has found that when patients use the guided imagery program, it results in shorter hospital stays and lower medical expenses.

Here is what the insurance company discovered during their initial study that brought about the practice of using meditation and visualization as support modalities for surgery:

Blue Shield of California studied 905 men and women who used guided imagery recordings in conjunction with surgeries, such as hysterectomies and cardiac procedures. Overall, those who listened to the recordings had a shorter hospital stay, lost less blood, used less pain medication, experienced fewer complications and saved Blue Shield $2,000 per patient in the study.[3]

While guided imagery and meditation can reduce stress, some of the other benefits noted in this study—less blood loss, less pain medication, and fewer complications—make a strong case that mind-body work can also influence our physiology.

USING MEDITATION
TO CALM THE STRESS RESPONSE

As outlined in chapter four, when we are stressed, it activates a series of physical responses in the body that are non-conducive to conception. This is why using meditation to reduce stress and remove these negative responses in our bodies can be one of the most powerful tools in promoting conception. Again, stress—whether it is originating from our old, unprocessed issues or coming from our day-to-day routine—is perhaps the most powerful detriment to fertility.

Dr. Deepak Chopra, in his book *Perfect Health: The Complete Mindbody Guide*, recommends using meditation techniques not only to reduce stress but to remove negative emotions in our bodies. Chopra discusses how stress hormones can be as damaging as chemical toxins in our bodies, and he explains how those toxins are the outcome of unresolved emotional issues:

Physical impurities in the cells have their equivalents in the mind: fear, anger, greed, compulsiveness, doubt and other negative emotions. Operating at the quantum level, they can be as damaging to us as any chemical toxin.... the mind-body connection turns negative attitudes into chemical toxins, the so-called "stress hormones" that have been linked to many different diseases.[4]

Chopra goes on to say that: "If properly taught and used, meditation allows a person to become unstuck from all of the ama [*ama* is the word Chopra uses for negative emotions] in his thoughts and emotions."[5]

So, meditation can be used to reduce stress. It can be used as a follow-up to session work, not only to process our toxic issues, but also to reprogram the subconscious. In meditation, as one enters the theta brain state or theta level of relaxation, it opens the door to communicate with the subconscious mind and enables us to do the follow-up work required to heal and overcome the unfavorable programming of the past. It is that deep level of relaxation that allows us to access the subconscious material. In a normal conscious or waking state, we are communicating primarily with the critical mind, and the work we do is unlikely to have any impact on the information buried in the subconscious. In other words, the power of a positive suggestion or affirmation used in meditation is far more powerful than when it is said in the waking state, because the part of the mind receiving that communication is the part where the changes need to take place.

Are there other ways that we can utilize meditation? Can we use meditation as a mind-body technique to heal ourselves?

MIND-BODY HEALING

Meditation, and the utilization of visualization techniques, opens the door to many possibilities in the realm of mind-body healing. I believe it can potentiate work that is being done in both Eastern and Western medical modalities, and I feel that this is one of the most valuable techniques that can be used in the fertility process. Mind-body healing is the process where an individual focuses on restoring physical harmony to their body, while in a meditative state. Some clients might use it to enhance Eastern medical modalities by strengthening the energy to the ovaries in order to help the follicles become stronger and more viable. Some will use mind-body healing to increase blood flow to the uterine lining. Others may employ mind-body healing to work with hormone levels or enhance ovulation, and others might use it around the time of a Western medical treatment, such as an IVF procedure, to support an embryo that has been transferred into the uterus. My belief is that mind-body work can be an invaluable part of healing, a method in which healing messages can be communicated to the cells (see chapter eight on cellular reprogramming), and a technique that can help each individual address issues that they feel might be blocking their fertility. Is there scientific proof that mind-body healing really works? More studies are needed, and many are underway. This book cites several studies in which the mind-body connection has proven to be beneficial. If it has been shown to be effective with other deficiencies in our bodies, why can't it be used specifically for healing and enhancing fertility?

I find that most women would much rather try to enhance their fertility by utilizing mind-body techniques than simply sit back, anxiously wait to see what will happen, and worry about bad news. If she does the mind-body work, a woman becomes an active participant in her fertility process; if not, she is simply an onlooker and often feels like a victim. In one situation, a woman feels empowered as she works with her body; in the other, she watches and waits for a miracle, perhaps a miracle of medicine. In one case, a woman is actively creating her future and her reality; in the other, she is passively observing. In the first scenario, a woman feels like she is doing everything she can to be successful; in the other, she may feel like a bystander in her own life, wondering if there was more that could have been done. Is it false hope, or is this a resource with a potential that, for the most part, has been unexplored?

I believe mind-body techniques can create a sense of empowerment in women who are seeking to understand and embrace their fertility. Frankly, there are no guarantees in fertility work, whether a patient is at the doctor's office undergoing IVF procedure or she is using meditation to try to visualize her body releasing healthy, viable follicles. Doesn't it make sense to somehow mobilize the body's innate resources?

In the end, perhaps the most important issue is whether or not the client feels that she has benefited from the process of utilizing meditation and mind-body healing. Most of the clients I see—supported by the case studies throughout this book—feel that the mind-body work helped them immensely. Whether it was learning how to achieve the relaxation response, how to send positive messages to their cells, how to release toxic thoughts, how to visualize and create a successful future, or how to do mind-body healing, it may not matter, as long as the process served them in a beneficial way. Additionally, the meditative tools learned on the fertility journey can be used for other life challenges long after their baby has arrived.

YOUR THOUGHTS CREATE YOUR FUTURE

It is has been said that every thought is a prayer, every belief is a prayer. By giving thoughts and beliefs time and energy, we are giving them life, almost as if we are praying for those things to occur. What we think, write, say, feel, or believe becomes our truth. We create our own reality—our thoughts manifest into what we see occurring in our lives. In other words, by thinking, worrying, verbalizing, or believing negative thoughts, we are giving those thoughts power, and that, in turn, shapes our destiny. Conversely, when we have a positive attitude and positive outlook, we open up to the possibility of a future that brings all of our dreams to life. Our thoughts, whether they are positive or negative, become part of our belief system, and this profoundly affects the events and experiences of our lives.

For example, the individual who introduces herself as a struggling businesswoman has defined her truth and her position in the business world. She will most likely continue to struggle as long as she expresses her identity in that manner. Conversely, if that same person has lots of excitement and energy about that business and believes her business will flourish and prosper, she creates an aura of success around her. Even if this is a new enterprise and she has only a few clients, as long as she introduces herself with enthusiasm about how the business is "growing and getting more exciting every day," she is mapping out her success. What we believe now will come to us in the future. That is why we are told to express gratitude for things we want to create even though they haven't yet appeared in our lives. It is a way of manifesting those things.

This concept, often referred to as the "Law of Attraction," has been around for centuries. It is considered a law of psychodynamics or thought, not a scientifically accepted law, although there are studies that claim it may have some quantitative validity. In its simplest form, it says *our thoughts, feelings, and beliefs create our destiny.*

So, it becomes important to look at what our thoughts, feelings, and beliefs are creating. If a woman who is trying to get pregnant is enmeshed in negative thoughts 90 percent of the time, what will her future be like? Thoughts like: "What if I never get pregnant and never get to experience being a mother?" "I've been trying so hard to become pregnant with all of the drugs and procedures, for such a long time, that I can't get myself to believe anymore." "It makes me too sad to even think about trying to have a baby after the miscarriage." "I don't know if I deserve to get pregnant because of my past," can have a profound effect on whether or not she achieves her goal.

An important consideration about the negative energy and negative self-talk we create is to acknowledge the source of that material, which is the programming within the subconscious mind. A woman may *consciously* be telling herself that she *will* get pregnant this cycle while her subconscious is overpowering that sentiment with fears or stress or guilt or feelings of inadequacy. As mentioned in chapter three, new research shows that the subconscious mind controls about 95 percent of what goes on in our lives, and the conscious mind only 5 percent. Which one is going to win that battle?

THE VISUALIZATION PROCESS

The case studies throughout this book have one common element. Each of the women was using meditation to visualize or create her future. I believe that when this work is done in the theta state—in meditation or hypnosis—it appears to have an enhanced power that helps overcome old subconscious programming and beliefs.

Subconscious work is always done in the present tense. If you do an affirmation in future tense that says, "I will have a prosperous business" or "I will get pregnant and have a baby," you are instructing the subconscious that it is okay to delay this work until some time in the future. What if that is ten years from now? Working in the present tense implies that you are actively making changes now, whereas future tense implies that this may be nothing more than a wish or a dream. If you want to change your reality with the subconscious mind, it should be approached as if the manifestation of what you desire is already in progress. People who believe in the law of attraction support this understanding because they *know* that the changes they wish to create in their lives are *already in place*.

Believing is also feeling. In fact, the feeling of gratitude experienced when one has manifested a desire is an essential part of the creation process. That means that in order to create a pregnancy, part of the work involves embracing the positive emotions of being pregnant and feeling gratitude for the pregnancy *before* conception has even taken place. The best way to lay the groundwork for this is to begin a daily meditation where the feelings of joy and excitement of being pregnant and perhaps even holding a new baby in your arms make you feel complete bliss and gratitude.

Psychotherapist and motivational speaker Dr. Wayne Dyer explains the importance of visualization in his book *Real Magic*:

> Learn to act as if the life you visualize were already here. Act as if that which you perceive in your mind were already here in the physical world. Begin treating your thoughts and visions as much more than simple amorphous meanderings of your mind. You create your thoughts, your thoughts create your intentions, your intentions create your reality.... start the practice of acting as if the images you desire were already your reality.[6]

Dyer encourages everyone to visualize as if what you want to manifest has *already happened*.

The law of attraction can produce whatever we desire. The key is to remember that the messages being communicated by the subconscious mind are what truly govern this process. If the subconscious is consumed with positive thoughts and beliefs, we can manifest our dreams. A subconscious mind that contains negative emotions is likely to produce frustration and failure.

THE FOUR STEPS OF MANIFESTATION

There are four phases or steps that can be used in meditation in order to manifest what we want to achieve.

1. The first part of manifesting the future is visualizing what we want to create.

2. The second part is to remove or process old subconscious programming that may be interfering or creating a far different picture than what we want to see coming to fruition. This step is probably the most important part of this process and yet it is the one that is often ignored. If old programs of fear or inadequacy or sadness or guardedness or any of a number of subconscious beliefs are present within our subconscious mind, that will block our ability to be in vibration with the things we want to manifest. In other words, until we work on our stuff, we cannot create what we want to generate in our lives because the deep-rooted feelings will interfere with this process. For example, someone can spend years imagining their perfect partner, but if they have a protective wall around them due to bad relationships in the past, that partner cannot come into being until the old issues and barriers have been removed and that person is fully open to receive a new relationship. People who think that manifestation is simply a matter of positive thinking—without doing the necessary internal work—are leaving out the most critical step in this process.

3. The third step in this process is embracing the feeling of joy for what we want to create, and that feeling should match the intensity we might get as if we had already manifested our goal. In other words, in the context of fertility, this means to capture and experience the feeling a woman would have when she held her baby for the first time.

4. A fourth part of the equation—according to the spiritual teachers—is to establish alignment or connection to whatever we be-

lieve is our source or spirit. While embracing that connection, we are to express gratitude for what is being created. This last step is a personal choice, and each individual can decide if that concept resonates with them and if they want to utilize their connection to their source to manifest a pregnancy. (There is more information about this in chapter ten.)

All four elements are key components of *attracting* what we want to manifest in our lives, and meditation is the best vehicle for carrying us through these steps.

MEDITATION ONE: FOR STRESS RELIEF

Close your eyes and take ten deep breaths. With each breath, bring more calmness and relaxation into your mind and body. Imagine that you are out in a beautiful place in nature. That can be any place that feels safe for you: the mountains, the beach, or just in a beautiful garden. Allow yourself to feel happy and at peace in your surroundings. If it feels okay to you, imagine that a gentle rain is starting to fall. If you don't like rain, then you can substitute the rays of the sun or even moonlight in place of rain. As the rain or moonlight or sun washes over you, allow yourself to let go of any stress or tension in your body. Stay with this image for about five minutes and allow nature to help you cleanse or wash off any tension that you might feel. Allow your mind and body to relax fully and completely.

When you are ready, take three deep breaths and gently open your eyes. Notice how your body feels. This is a meditation that you can use every day for stress reduction.

MEDITATION TWO: VISUALIZING YOUR FUTURE

The following meditation is a practical exercise putting the law of attraction into action. If it elicits an emotional response, don't be surprised. That is a fairly common response. A discussion of the significance of the emotions that might arise appears right after the meditation.

Close your eyes and take ten slow, deep breaths, breathing all the way down to the bottom of your lungs. Each time you exhale, allow yourself to relax a little more.

Imagine yourself in the future. Imagine that you are at home, feeling very safe and comfortable, looking at your body in the mirror. Notice that you are about seven months along in your pregnancy, and seeing your round belly creates a feeling of joy. The shape and curves of your body may look a little different, but there is incredible beauty in your pregnant body. Notice the overwhelming sense of joy and gratitude you feel after doing all of the positive work that made this possible. Stay with those images for a few minutes and understand that this is who you are and what you are creating.

Imagine a few more months have passed and you are holding your newborn baby. Imagine the warmth of the baby's body next to yours. Enjoy the moment of closeness and connection. Experience the wonderful joy and gratitude as this becomes a preview of what is already in motion in your life. Hold these feelings for a few minutes and take ownership of your future. From this point forward, choose this as your reality.

When you are ready, count up from one to ten, allowing more awareness to come in with each number you count, and then gently open your eyes. It is beneficial to write down your thoughts and feelings after this exercise.

EMOTIONAL RESPONSES

If there are intense feelings and/or negative emotions that interfere with being able to do the "visualizing your future" meditation, know that you aren't alone. Many women will discover that subconscious issues might make this meditation a difficult experience. If you find that, during this exercise, there are doubts, fears, sadness, or interfering negative thoughts, it is usually an indication that work still needs to be done to process and heal the old subconscious material. Remember, an essential part of conception is clearing out the negative information in the subconscious mind which is, in evvect, putting a wall between you and your ability to have a baby.

The other important consideration about any negative thoughts that may have come up in this exercise is to look closely at how those very thoughts may be what you are *visualizing* or creating as part of your future. In other words, questioning whether you will ever get pregnant or have a child indicates the type of energy that surrounds this process as *you* shape your reality. Your doubts or fears or possible feelings of inadequacy become the truth in your life. Are you creating a journey where pregnancy comes easily because you are in a place of knowing and believing in yourself, or are you overwhelmed by fear and doubt, and unable to create what you really want?

This meditation is a valuable tool because it can sometimes help us discover whether or not there are issues that are blocking conception, or it can become a powerful way of shaping what we want to create in life. The important thing to know is that even if the feelings that came up were negative, those subconscious issues can be processed and healed. We can all take charge of shaping our future.

In Their Own Words

At age forty-one, Karen opted to use an IVF procedure to get pregnant. Like all women working on infertility, Karen had some issues that were interfering with her ability to conceive, including financial concerns and what it would be like if she stepped away from the workforce to raise a child. The other major issue for Karen was her age. According to the ART Report, a woman in her age group has only an 12 percent chance of having a baby if she undergoes in vitro using her own eggs.

Karen used meditation and visualization to manifest what she wanted to create. At one key point in her journey—documented in her account—she experienced a major shift. At that moment, everything came together. The subconscious mind was free of blocks, and suddenly Karen was able to really visualize her future. From that point forward, there was no doubt about her success.

Karen's Story
Creating a Miracle

I met my husband when I was thirty-six years old and we married shortly after I turned thirty-eight. Mine was a classic case of "not meeting the right one at the right time" until later in life. I was on birth control pills for ten years prior to marrying my husband, and stopped taking them about three months before our wedding. I was terrified that I would get pregnant in those three months and be unable to wear my very fitted wedding dress. Little did I know!

Needless to say, no unexpected pregnancy happened and we waltzed through our wedding and off to Hawaii where I was certain (again) that we would be pregnant and have a "honeymoon" baby nine months following our nuptials. No pregnancy. We took no precautions and had a lot of fun for the next six to seven months. Still no results.

In the meantime, I began to worry—ever so slightly—about a past diagnosis of endometriosis and my age. At twenty-eight I'd gone through a laparoscopy for endometriosis. I'd had terrible periods and cramps in my youth that got worse and worse until I was missing work every month due to the pain and nausea. After the surgery I went on the pill and never had a problem or hardly even a cramp again. I'd totally forgotten about it until we weren't getting pregnant. Suddenly, it began to gnaw at the back of my mind... what if that were the problem? My age began to worry me as well.

I'd grown up in an era where women could have it all—a career, love, children, everything—and it didn't seem to matter when you started on the children part. I saw celebrities well into their late forties having kids, and thought nothing of it. Now, I know that they probably had a medical intervention to accomplish this feat. So about seven months after the wedding we went to the one and only infertility doctor on our insurance list. He immediately scheduled another laparoscopy for the prior-diagnosed endometriosis and assured us that was the problem.

One month later I had the surgery, followed by horrid complications. This set us back another five to six months and also sent us running to a very respected and well-known infertility group—costs be damned. We weren't going to put our future dreams in the hands of a discount doctor. We went through their medical workup and a couple of IUIs before we first heard the words "in vitro" used in respect to our situation. I grew up knowing of Louise Brown, the test-tube baby, but never, ever dreamed that I would one day be looking at that as an option for having my own child.

Unfortunately, none of the lower-tech solutions worked for us so we marched on into in vitro with heads held high and fears at bay. Four to five shots a day (some of them done while I cried and looked the other way), patches, suppositories, pills, almost daily doctor's appointments—it was all so *medical*, but we were determined to do it right and succeed.

Almost one year to the day after the laparoscopic surgery for the endometriosis, we were back in the operating room, but this time for a suspected tubal pregnancy and a D and C (dilation and curettage procedure). We were successful—sort of. We'd gotten pregnant, but that pregnancy wasn't progressing right—a blighted ovum as they called it, and the doctors feared that another embryo had implanted on one of my tubes. Thankfully, they were wrong about the tubal pregnancy, but still no baby!

Suddenly this was not fun any more. We decided to stop the madness for a bit. We wanted to have fun again. We wanted to laugh and play and do it the old-fashioned way. So we did. We took a year off. We traveled. We went out. We had parties. But still, we wanted a baby. And we tried to get pregnant with every old wives' tale in the book. If someone mentioned that they'd gotten pregnant by drinking Robitussin, we drank it. If someone else got pregnant by putting their legs up afterward, we held ours up for an hour, laughing the whole time. If someone else got pregnant the minute they started adoption procedures ... well, we weren't ready for that ... yet. But we did start discussing adoption—tentatively.

A year later the company where I worked announced plans to close the office. We decided to give in vitro one last try. The doctors did the tests again, checking to make sure that my eggs were still viable—fortunately, they were, although I was forty-one years old by now. I did not take the promotion with my company but the severance instead. Two months after my company closed up shop and I was not working (for the first time since I was fourteen years old), we were back into shots and pills and doctor's appointments. But this time we also tried some alternative things, including hypnosis.

I honestly believe that hypnosis was one of the major factors in making this second in vitro successful! I was older. I was worried about not working and the financial concerns that go along with that. I had so many tapes playing in my head about how I was too old, too late, too this, too that—that it would never work. We were three years into this and gone were those naïve and hopeful thoughts of getting pregnant and not fitting into a wedding dress. I believed that it would take a miracle for this to work. And miracles didn't seem to happen to me ... only to other people. Or that's what I thought.

I knew enough now from my hours and hours of internet research that an older woman's chances of getting pregnant get slimmer and slimmer with each passing year or month or day or even hour. At that time I could only picture my eggs shriveling and wilting every minute, until they resembled forlorn little raisins sitting idly in my body, unable to muster the energy to meet up with their sperm boyfriends in the tubes or even in a petri dish. My hypnotherapist worked with me on so many levels to help me visualize the eggs growing, my body responding, the baby growing, our future unfolding. It was possible.

I remember one meditation in particular where I looked into the future at our baby's first birthday party. I *saw* it! I really did.

With each passing session, I became so certain that it could work—that my body could work! Age be damned. The internet and all of the research be damned. I went into hypnotherapy a bit of a skeptic. Obviously, I was willing to try anything, but the funny thing was ... I started to really believe in it! I would do the meditations, and I really could *see* the eggs growing. I could see the embryos becoming strong and healthy. I could see them attaching and dividing and taking a strong hold. I could *see* it. I mean really, really *see* it. I told my husband about it. I asked him to lie in bed with me and we'd do the meditations together ... he's a very analytical, cerebral, realistic attorney so this was a true testament of his love and desire. We did it together, as we did the shots and the doctor's appointments and the medical rigmarole as well. But it was the hypnosis sessions that made me skip lightly as I left ... and made me *believe*.

There were a couple of issues that loomed large in my subconscious—the financial implications of not working and staying home to care for our baby, and the issue of my age. I got my first job at the age of fourteen and had worked my way through college into teaching and then into the corporate world, so it was strange indeed to think of not working. But my husband and I also knew that we didn't want to have a baby and then have someone else take care of this baby as we both went to work. It was understood that I would stay home and care for our children while he worked.

It seems so traditional and almost un-hip to say that these days, but he would be the breadwinner, and I would be the homemaker (at least through the first few years of our future children's lives). But I think that there was some deep-rooted fear involved in this for me. I had never had anyone take care of me before—at least not as an adult. I hadn't been dependent on anyone since I left high school.

Somehow this desired pregnancy also carried a bit of fear and uncertainty with it. I would have to put my faith in someone else to take care of me and this baby. It was a scary vision for someone who didn't really trust anyone but herself to take care of things. We worked on this in hypnosis and uprooted some very far-reaching fears from my childhood and early adulthood. I had struggled financially in my early adulthood and knew the stress of not being able to pay bills while in college. But if I got pregnant and we had a baby, I knew I didn't want to work. It was such a conundrum and certainly it wreaked havoc with my subconscious. The mind-body work helped me to visualize the future where the baby would be clothed and we wouldn't be rolling the dice because baby needs new shoes.

This fear had nothing to do with my husband and his ability to provide … it was a deep-rooted, emotionally charged issue from *my* past. But it had to be dealt with on some level before my body could respond to the pregnancy issue. Also, by this time, my age had become a huge, gnarling issue … one that played in my head continually. I had by now gained a lot of internet information and misinformation that made me fear each passing day as an obstacle to our baby. I was *old*; I told myself that almost daily. I had always looked much younger than my actual years and always felt even younger. I had always loved my birthdays, even looked forward to them. They were celebrations! But suddenly birthdays became something to dread. I would look in the mirror and see this haggard old creature, surely unable to produce viable eggs.

We worked on this in a way where I, once again, became the strong and vibrant person who not only hiked and snowshoed in the mountains, but who also was healthy and had strong and viable eggs. Once again, I had confidence in my body and its abilities. I was confident! I was happy. I knew that my body could do this. And it did.

As I type this, our fifteen-month-old daughter is talking to herself in her crib upstairs. She is the most beautiful, precious thing in our lives. I am not working. I stay home with her every day, and we are not living on skid row. We have a life that I only dreamed of once upon a time. Although there are days where I envy my husband's ability to go to meet with clients and have fancy lunches that don't include renditions of "The Itsy Bitsy Spider" or baby meltdowns of biblical proportions, I wouldn't trade it for the world!

Almost every day, I say thank you … out loud … for the gift of our daughter. To me, hypnotherapy was one of the major reasons that it worked—along with modern medical interventions. I believe now, more than ever, that the *things* you tell yourself subconsciously—that you believe—have such a significant influence on outcomes. And you don't even know it most of the time. Hypnotherapy helped me to address my issues and then reinvent the story, the outcome, the future into the one I have. I was able to *see* what I wanted and to visualize it through meditations.

And then the future came … she was born early at only five pounds, but the weight of her *being* has changed us in ways I am unable to articulate accurately … and there are times now that when I see her, my heart breaks just a little with the love that I feel. I would go through it all again a million times over just to have her.

Those hypnotherapy sessions have had a continual effect on my life. Even now when I feel fear creeping in, I visualize what I want. I meditate. I try to create a new tape recording within myself … and it works.

WORKS CITED

1. Herbert Benson, *The Relaxation Response* (New York: Harper Collins Publishers, 2000), quoted in Joel Stein, "Just Say Om," *Time Magazine* (Aug. 4, 2003).

2. Ibid.

3. Polly Drew, "A Guided Journey to Peace," *Compass* (April 17, 2005). http://www.redorbit.com/news/health/144522/compass_polly_drew_a_guided_journey_to_peace/index.html.

4. Deepak Chopra, *Perfect Health: The Complete Mind-body Guide* (New York: Harmony Books, 1991), 122.

5. Ibid.

6. Wayne Dyer, *Real Magic* (New York: Harper Collins Publishers, 1992), 81.

CHAPTER TEN

ENERGY WORK:
Healing at the Core

We are intellectual beings. When people make the decision to work on their issues, they usually want to reach an understanding of why things occurred the way they did. They want to know what happened and why people behaved in ways that not only defied logic but also defied our basic understanding of right and wrong. It is fairly common for people to start this process by talking through their issues in an attempt to find clarity. This first step can be very beneficial, but it may not always bring the completion we need. Sometimes we try to do all of our healing and processing above the shoulders and neglect the feelings that are stuck in our bodies. In other words, we try to intellectualize the negative events that have occurred in our lives. While it is beneficial to have a logical understanding and clarity about our issues, the negative energy—directly related to those emotional issues—can remain stuck in our physical bodies. Processing and removing that negative energy helps us to not only reach an emotional state of well-being, but it also frees the body of divisive obstructions that can interfere with our physical health by disrupting the flow of the healthy energy within our physiology.

Our bodies are made up of energy. In the practice of Eastern medicine, acupuncture is based on the movement of *chi* or life force energy that flows through our bodies along channels called *meridians*. Despite resistance in the past from some in the Western medical community, the existence of meridians and the flow of energy has now been well documented. It has also been established that there is a direct relationship between the quality of our physical health and our body's ability to maintain an even flow of energy through all of our meridians. Conversely, disruptions in the flow of that healthy energy can create physical disharmonies.

While much of this book has focused on mental and emotional healing, I believe our issues have physical and energetic counterparts that can create disharmonies in our physiology. In other words, an emotional issue from our past might show up in our physical body in a couple of ways: it can become a barrier or block to the healthy flow of chi or it can settle into a weak area of our body and form an uncomfortable energetic mass or disturbance. For example, when someone gets fearful or anxious, they often report feeling a knot in their stomach. Is this knot an actual physical abnormality, or could it be coming from an energetic memory that has been festering there for years? What about the person who feels tightness in their chest and has difficulty breathing each time they experience stress? Could this be a stress response that may have begun years ago when an emotional event causing distress lodged itself in a vulnerable part of the body? Practitioners of Chinese medicine and energy healers often see clients who report having taken themselves to emergency rooms because their physical symptoms were so strong and frightening they believed they were in crisis, yet all their tests were negative and they were left feeling confused and frustrated by a lack of diagnosis. Clearly they did not just imagine their discomfort. Whether on a large scale such as this, or on a smaller scale such as the nervous stomach, we have all experienced examples of how energy blocks occur in the body and manifest as real physical discomforts.

Dr. Christiane Northrup, in her book *Women's Bodies, Women's Wisdom*, made this observation about how emotional energy can manifest in our bodies:

> Mental and emotional energy goes in and out of physical form regularly, bouncing on the continuum between energy and matter, particle and wave. Quite simply, emotional and mental energy can become physical in our bodies.[1]

Northrup goes on to say that the act of healing takes place on many levels: "True healing, not just curing our body or soothing our mental anxiety, involves transformation of our energy field and consciousness."[2] The process of healing is a multilevel transformation because it involves the physical, mental, emotional, and energetic dimensions.

When a negative emotional signal is communicated to the physical body, it can cause a block or disturbance in the flow of healthy chi which, in turn, can create a physical disharmony. Energy healer and psychotherapist Barbara Brennan, in her book, *Hands of Light*, says that "energy blocks lead eventually to physical disorder."[3] These energetic disharmonies and subsequent physical disorders can include breakdowns in the body's ability to conceive. For example, an energetic block in the abdomen might cut off the flow of healthy chi to the ovaries. If the ovaries are depleted of their healthy energy, they won't be able to enrich or nurture the follicles, and, of course, viable follicles are a necessity for conception to occur. On a positive note, Brennan believes that when we process and heal our blocks, it promotes the circulation of healthy chi, which, in turn, opens the doors for us to manifest what we want to create in life. "When we begin releasing our blocks, we do our personal task.... By clearing away your personal blocks, you pave the way to accomplish your deepest longing."[4] Thus, when we address the emotional and energetic issues, we remove the physical blocks and allow conception—the "deepest longing" for many of the readers of this book—to take place.

Since this concept might be new to a lot of people, it might be helpful to look at this in a more personal way. Try doing this meditation and pay very careful attention to reactions in your physical body.

MEDITATION

For this meditation, you can either go back to times in your life when events like this actually occurred, or just imagine these things happening. The key to this meditation is making it seem like you are really there and tuning in to the feelings and emotions in your body.

Part A

Imagine that you are at the doctor's office. You and your husband are waiting to hear about the tests that were performed to determine why you haven't been able to get pregnant. Having a child is something you've wanted all of your life, and you can't understand why this has become so hard. As you wait, fears about not being able to have children race through your mind. Finally, when the doctor comes into the room, her expression is one of disappointment. When you hear the news—the chances of having a baby with your own eggs are less than 5 percent—you can feel those words resonate through your body. You look over at your husband and can see that he is trying to hide his disappointment. You feel like you are letting everyone down. *Check in with your body. If you feel stress, where is it located in your body? Is there a tightness in your chest? Difficulty breathing? An elevated heart rate? A knot in your stomach? A jittery feeling running through your body? Really connect with your body to feel what is happening.*

Part B

A couple months later, after you have undergone a procedure such as an IUI or IVF and felt that this cycle was *the one*, you discover that you've started your period. You rack your brain for something positive to tell yourself, but you feel like you are out of ideas. You feel defeated and find yourself wondering if this is a punishment for something you did in the past. In a brief moment of panic, the thought of "how am I going to tell everyone" comes into your mind. *Check in with your body. If you feel stress, where is it located in your body? Is there a tightness in your chest? Difficulty breathing? An elevated heart rate? A knot in your stomach? A jittery feeling running through your body? Really connect with your body and feel what is happening.*

Part C

It is the following night, and you are at a small gathering with family members. Everyone wants to know how things went with your cycle. All eyes are on you, waiting for your response. The pressure feels intense, and part of you just wants to run away. You wish you'd never mentioned the procedure to anyone. After you tell them that the procedure failed, someone tries to comfort you with the last thing you want to hear: "You can always adopt." Everyone tries to be understanding, but you internalize the looks on their faces as "you've let us down again." *Check in with your body. If you feel stress, where is it located in your body? Is there a tightness in your chest? Difficulty breathing? An elevated heart rate? A knot in your stomach? A jittery feeling running through your body? Really connect with your body and feel what is happening.*

Take a moment, open your eyes and write down all of the physical responses in your body. When that is complete, it is important to clean away these negative thoughts and feelings.

Part D

Close your eyes again and imagine that you are taking a shower and washing away all of the negative thoughts and feelings that came up in this meditation. After you feel cleansed and rejuvenated, take a moment and imagine that you are stepping out into a sunny, fertile garden. As you breathe in the surroundings of that garden, bring that fertile energy into your body. Know that the meditation you just did was simply designed to help you understand a concept and that it is in no way a reflection of you or your future. As you read this book and work on your issues, you are transforming—much like an emerging butterfly—and getting more and more in touch with your fertile body. Know that your fertile body is coming into alignment with your desires. All of the work you are doing now is preparing your body for conception. Allow yourself to absorb the nurturing energy of this fertile garden and bring that energy into your body.

WHERE DID YOU FEEL THE RESPONSE?

How did you feel during each part of that meditation? What did you feel in your physical body? That meditation was designed to tap into several issues that might elicit emotional responses. It may have brought up the issues of "am I good enough" or "am I worthy." It may have tapped into perfectionism or fear of failure. It may have created feelings of rejection. It may have brought up anxiety or conjured up earlier times when you didn't know how to speak up or defend yourself.

Were those feelings in your logical *mind*, or were they occurring in your physical *body*? For most people, the responses were *felt* in the physical body. And for a lot of people, those feelings were very familiar and had been present on many occasions in the past. This is because the meditation was tapping into old emotional energies and issues that are still residing in the body. Noticing our responses on a visceral level tells us how we hold our emotions in our bodies. While this concept may seem a little out there to some people, the feelings in the body are very real. We can choose to ignore negative sensations in the body, but in doing so, we often end up feeling them over and over and living with them for a lifetime. We can choose to attend to those feelings and heal them at their source, and by doing that, we open the way for more positive feelings of happiness, joy, and inner peace to become part of our being.

If we don't address and heal the source of our negative responses, can this affect the body's ability to conceive? The answer to that question may lie in one of the physical responses that the majority of women experience when they participate in this chapter's meditation. Most people respond to the scenarios of the meditation with uncomfortable feelings in the *abdominal* area. It is very doubtful that the knot or queasiness in the abdomen is a brand new sensation and was felt for the first time during this meditation. This is probably a response that has occurred many times throughout life. It may have become a predictable reaction with an origin or source that goes back to when we were very young.

An example of this is a woman who feels like she is unworthy, not meeting expectations, or letting people down. That feeling of not being good enough could have come initially from the rejection by a parent, a sibling, a teacher, a lover, or even a group of friends. Every disappointment or rejection since that time compounds or reinforces that wound, triggering that same uncomfortable feeling at our energetic core.

What does this tell us? The emotional energy of not being good enough—which originated from an earlier life experience—is still present in that woman's body. Every time that woman has her menstrual period after a failed procedure or a cycle in a month where it had looked like it might finally be successful, those feelings of despair, inadequacy, or unworthiness return and hit with full force. Unworthiness is a common reaction to a situation where we have felt rejection in the past. Even if we have discovered, *on an intellectual level*, that worthiness is an issue in our lives, it is very likely that the negative energy connected to that might still reside somewhere in our bodies.

NEGATIVE ENERGY AND CONCEPTION

I believe that negative energy in our physiology can have a harmful effect on the body's receptivity to pregnancy and the reproductive process. How could that be possible? Imagine a mass of negative energy (created by many fearful thoughts and beliefs about fertility) taking the shape of a large abdominal tumor that is sucking all the life force and nutrients out of the reproductive system. As it drains the healthy energy, it is also blocking or robbing the flow of chi to the ovaries, and without their positive energetic charge, the ovaries are unable to produce viable follicles. Maybe that energetic tumor is creating a weakness where the body becomes unable to produce the proteins necessary for an embryo to implant in the uterus. Maybe that ball of negative energy is festering and promoting the spread of endometriosis. Maybe the unhealthy growth is draining the flow of chi to the uterus and as a consequence, the uterus is unable to support an embryo for a prolonged period of time. Maybe it is obstructing and restricting the uterine blood flow. If those outcomes, described above, were the result of a *physical* tumor instead of an *energetic* tumor, most people would be very understanding of the resultant symptomology. How do we know that an energetic tumor can't create the same results? How do we know that the knot or sick feeling in the gut that so many people experience isn't having a similar negative effect on the physical body?

Some skeptics in the scientific community might want to dismiss any relationship between energy within the body and physical health, but this isn't a new idea that is going to go away soon. Eastern medicine—which has been practiced successfully for 5,000 years—is based on working with the energy within our bodies. There is also a huge population of world-wide practitioners who specialize in what is known as energy work or energy healing. While this concept might be new to some readers, the practice of working with energy to promote physical healing is utilized every day by tens of thousands of practitioners around the world. After all, if our bodies are made up of atoms—which are comprised of protons, electrons, and neutrons—doesn't that suggest that energy might play some part in the functionality of our bodies? We can choose to honor or ignore the feelings in our bodies, but the mental, emotional, physical, and energetic all work together to make up our total health picture—all of these elements create who we are. Based on my experience in this area, I feel that the negative energies or blocks in our bodies—an outgrowth of our emotional issues—*do* have an adverse effect on our physical health. Until an issue is resolved and released on an emotional *and* energetic level, it is still part of who we are and has a profound influence on the inner workings of our physiology.

LOOKING AT ENERGY FROM A DIFFERENT PERSPECTIVE

The concept of negative energy creating blocks in our bodies may be new and different enough that it might be difficult for some to embrace. So let's look at it from a different perspective.

Imagine a woman who is trying to get pregnant. Let's say that she has unresolved issues with her mother, and she is giving away 10 percent of her energy to that conflict. In other words, every time she has words with her mother, feels controlled by her mother, or gets upset or worried about her mother, it takes away 10 percent of her physical energy. (We all have experienced exhaustion after a period of worry or upset or frustration or feeling manipulated. That exhaustion is the result of us giving up or losing the energy that we invested in that conflict.) In addition to the mother issue, imagine that same woman also has difficulty with her controlling boss and gives up another 10 percent of her energy to that dynamic. Maybe she has unresolved emotional residue from a relationship with an ex-boyfriend or ex-husband and gives away 10 percent energetically to those old feelings she is trying to forget. Perhaps there is an in-law with a physical issue or a situation like alcoholism and 10 percent goes to her concern about that person. Maybe 10 percent of her energy goes into worrying about her husband's job; perhaps his job security or his unhappiness with the situation. Energy could also be going to a miscarriage, an old physical injury from an accident, a sibling who was always the favorite of her parents, and so on.

When everything is added up, that woman might be giving away 70–80 percent of her energy. That leaves her only 20–30 percent for creating healthy follicles, maintaining a rich uterine blood flow, and numerous other physical functions that are instrumental in creating fertility. If that woman is trying to conceive when she is a little older, will her body be able to reproduce when it is running at only 20–30 percent of capacity? She might be able to get away with that at age eighteen, but if she is forty-two, that energy is vital to her success.

While looking at the energy deficiencies in this context might help us get a different perspective about our body energetics, the bottom line is to evaluate the way we are distributing our energy and make changes if it is not available to the body for purposes of creating life. So, if an individual finds that they are feeling unappreciated, empty, and exhausted, there is a possibility it might be the physical energy they are giving away.

WHAT IS ENERGY WORK
AND WHY IS IT IMPORTANT?

Energy work can take many shapes and forms. It can include modalities such as acupuncture, where the practitioner is helping maintain an even flow of energy to all parts of the body, or hands-on healing and working with chakras. For the purposes of this chapter we are talking about maintaining a healthy flow of chi and/or removing negative energy blocks. Some modalities are designed to do this work, while others are not. One might go out and get a relaxing massage—which is working with the body in a wonderful, nurturing way—and while that bodywork is beneficial, it isn't designed to address emotional or energetic imbalances. Conversely, if that person is getting some deep tissue massage, and when the therapist touches a certain part of their body it elicits an emotional response, that may open the door to working with the corresponding issue. At that point, the issue could be addressed and processed, as long as the practitioner is able to provide the guidance needed to facilitate the healing process.

Modalities for this type of work may include reiki, hands-on healing, Qi Gong healing, and some types of deep tissue massage. In some cases, the process may simply be referred to as "energy work."

Dr. Caroline Myss refers to this work as "energy medicine." In her book, *Sacred Contracts,* Myss discusses the relationship between energy and healing:

> Energy medicine is a timeless method of healing. Its effectiveness ... comes from activating or freeing blocked energy that has accrued over time. These healing methods seek to break down heavy energy from the past to facilitate the flow of current energy. By healing and releasing negative attitudes and beliefs and traumatic memories that are pulling your energy into the past, you return that energy to the present time, where it enhances the vibration of your entire system.[5]

Myss focuses much of the emphasis for energy healing on working with the body's chakra system—the seven energy centers in our bodies (see figure 10.1). The "seven centers are like an energy spinal cord through which the life force, or prana, flows into our physical body. Each one represents a different configuration of physical, emotional, and psychological concerns."[6] If these centers are unbalanced, blocked, or releasing too much energy, it can indicate an emotional imbalance and result in corresponding physical disharmonies in the body.

Working with the chakra system and the energetics of our bodies has been practiced in many cultures throughout history. Chakras are cone-shaped centers of energy that are present in all of us. The word "chakra" means wheel or circle; chakras are typically described as spinning vortices of energy. The base or root of the energetic vortex is attached to the physical body, and the cone of the whirlwind becomes wider as it gets farther away from the body. All of the chakras enter the

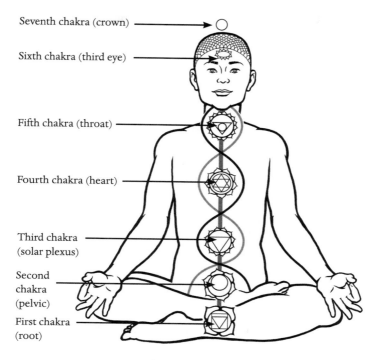

Seventh chakra (crown)

Sixth chakra (third eye)

Fifth chakra (throat)

Fourth chakra (heart)

Third chakra
(solar plexus)

Second
chakra
(pelvic)

First chakra
(root)

Figure 10.1: The body's chakra system.

body and connect to what Myss refers to as an energetic *spinal cord* that runs through the body. Most practitioners focus their healing work on what are considered to be the seven major chakras or energy centers.

If we look at the purpose of each of the chakras, starting from the lower chakras and working up the body to the top of the head, it is easy to see the relationship between these energy centers and physical and emotional traits that define who we are.

The first chakra, located at the bottom of the spine, is our connection to the earth. People who are described as being grounded or love spending time outdoors usually have strong energy in their first chakra, also referred to as the root chakra.

The second chakra governs the sexual and reproductive organs. I will talk about that chakra more in a moment, because that is the energy center that is connected to fertility.

The third chakra is connected to the area of the solar plexus. This chakra is associated with our courage and self-esteem. We feel many of our issues, like criticism, here because this energy center is the receptor site where we take in stimuli that can enhance or threaten our self-concept. When people talk about the "feeling in their gut," this energy center is where we experience those physical sensations.

The fourth chakra is the heart chakra. People who are loving and compassionate have vibrant heart chakras. One often feels a very open and accepting energy when they are in the presence of someone whose heart energy is dynamic and full of life.

The fifth chakra is the throat chakra. This energy center governs our ability to speak up and express our feelings. Individuals who were never allowed to speak up will often have weak energy in their throat chakra and consequently speak with very soft voices.

The sixth chakra is called the third eye. It is located in the middle of the forehead. The third eye is often represented in the art work of the ancient Egyptians. This is the intuitive energy center. It is a gateway to wisdom and intellect. People who are intuitives or seers use this chakra to absorb or bring in information.

The seventh or crown chakra is about our relationship to spiritual or Divine energy. It is the connection to God or Source or Creator, or whatever concept fits into one's belief system.

It is believed that the majority of the energy that supports our life force, also referred to as prana, enters our bodies primarily through the crown chakra, and through the root chakra, although each energy center has the ability to bring in or absorb essence or energy. Each of the chakras is a spinning vortex of energy. The healing objective when working with the chakras is to ensure that each of the channels of energy is open, vibrant, rotating in the proper direction, and receiving and moving energy through the body. After entering a trance state, some healers sense or *feel* chakras while others often *see* the chakras, each of which emits a different color. Through the use of certain specialized types of photography, the chakra energies have been photographed, observed, and recorded.

The second chakra, located a couple of inches below the belly button, is the energy center that relates to the reproductive organs. When this energy is healthy and flowing, the reproductive organs can function at their full capacity. However, if there is a block or disturbance in the second chakra, the energy needed to achieve full reproductive functioning may not be available to those organs. In theory, it is much like the healing philosophy in Eastern medicine: if the energy isn't reaching the desired organs, disharmony or underperformance can result. An example of this might be ovaries that are unable to generate or release viable follicles because they need more prana or life force energy to perform that function. Again, it is similar to acupuncture in that both systems are about balancing energy within our bodies and connecting us with external energy from the universe. While Western medicine will use drugs in an attempt to clinically increase the body's performance, energy medicine attempts to rectify the problem by correcting the energetic disharmonies.

Some of the things that might block or shut down the energy flow to the second chakra might include occurrences such as miscarriages, abortions, rape, betrayal, sexual abuse, or sexual mistrust from an old partner. Sometimes these issues also impact the level of sexual trust or openness that a woman is able to achieve. In other words, if a woman has negative feelings about her sexuality, it might be reflected as second chakra blockages connected to unresolved emotional issues. The way this affects the second chakra is to essentially shut it down so that it can't pull in or vibrate with energy. If the second chakra ceases to function properly, then it can create an infertile situation because there is no energy source to nourish the reproductive organs. When this area of the body shuts down, it can not only become unreceptive to lovemaking but also unreceptive to creating life. It should be noted that people who are caretakers are often giving away too much energy from—and drastically weakening—the second chakra. In some women, there appears to be a connection between giving away too much energy to caretaking and a variety of gynecological issues, including infertility.

Emotional issues are connected to the performance of the chakras. When these energy centers are not performing correctly, it is often a reflection of aspects of our personal history that have gone unprocessed.

THOSE WHO FEEL NOTHING

There are people who have shut down their emotions as a coping mechanism. There may have been some readers who emerged from the meditation experience at the beginning of this chapter and exclaimed that they didn't feel a thing. About 5 percent of the clients I see report that they don't experience emotions, or they only cry about every five or six years. This situation often indicates that they may have—at some point in their life—turned off their ability to feel. Perhaps this has come as a result of not being allowed to show emotions as a child or being in situations that were so uncomfortable that the accompanying feelings were too painful or emotional to bear. Experiencing emotions for some individuals can mean a loss of control and bring up feelings of vulnerability.

Being in a state of non-feeling indicates that this individual has disassociated from the ability to be in touch with emotions related to their issues. This adds an extra healing step to the process. First, that person will need to reconnect with their feelings before they can process those feelings. It is often difficult to get a client to reconnect with their feelings because, on a deep level, they really don't want to do that. They may have found a protective mechanism through their intellect that has served them for decades. It is important to emphasize that turning off the emotions does not mean that issues are not there: denial is not a form of healing. This is a person who has an extra step to go through before they can process the negative energies in their bodies.

I often find that women who come in feeling nothing benefit greatly by reconnecting with their emotions. After reestablishing this connection, they become much better parents because they have the ability to share emotions and feelings with their children. If the mother has switched off her feelings, how can the child learn to feel? How can a baby get a read on her mother's feelings if mother is surrounded by a protective wall? I have discovered that many women who want children almost always have to first regain some level of their own ability to feel.

WHERE TO GO FOR ENERGY WORK

In chapter thirteen, I talk about how to go about finding a healer. It helps to get referrals from people who have worked with practitioners specializing in energy work. It is more difficult to find a healer in this area because this calls for someone who can guide you through the processing of the emotional issues while also helping release the physical manifestations of those concerns. I combine hypnosis and energy work because I feel that healing the mind and body requires both modalities. As a rule, however, most hypnotists do not include energy work in their practice. In the future, we may see more therapists working together to facilitate this process. In other words, a psychotherapist might work on the emotional processing at the same time as an energy worker is releasing blocks in the physical body. If no referrals are available, it is a good idea to interview a couple of practitioners who do this work in order to find the person who feels right for you. For some people, finding and working with the right healer may mean traveling to another geographic location. If the results of this work are life-changing, as they often are, it might well be worth the cost of the trip.

In Their Own Words

Even though most of these accounts don't mention it by name, I use energy work with the majority of my clients. One way of knowing when the body energetics are in a healthy balance is by observing the receptivity the client experiences when introducing new dynamics—such as conceiving or carrying a baby—into the physical paradigm. In Catherine's story, it is easy to see how receptive her mind and body became to supporting and welcoming donor eggs. That was an indication that the negative energy had been cleared, leaving the mind and body open to visualizing and embracing a positive future.

Catherine's Story
The Mind-Body Connection

My history of infertility was brief compared to other women. I started trying to conceive at age forty-two. I got pregnant, but miscarried at five weeks. We did tests, and the good news was that every test they did was great: on a scale of 1 to 10, I had a ten in all of the tests except that I had a high FSH level because of my age. My FSH was 14–15, and then 16–17 after the Clomid challenge. So, we tried to do an IVF, but the cycle was cancelled because I only produced one good egg. That's when we opted for donor eggs. However, we would try to conceive via IUI over the next several months while we waited to get matched with a donor.

So, that is when I started hypnosis. Thinking it would take at least six months to get matched, I was surprised when it only took three weeks! While my chances to get pregnant increased with a donor egg, I was still very interested in what we were doing in hypnotherapy because I wanted to maximize my chances. Getting pregnant is an inexact science, and I wanted to increase my odds. Fortunately, except for my age, I didn't have any other physical issues working against me.

I was thrilled to get matched so quickly, but so surprised! I could be pregnant in just two months! In hypnosis, I wanted to create the warmest, healthiest, safest, and most loving environment to welcome my embryos. So, we worked on being accepting of using donor embryos and getting my mind and body totally calm and peaceful for a healthy and full-term pregnancy.

Hypnosis helped me in various ways. First, it was very, very relaxing. I literally could feel so much positive energy within me. We did some mind-body cellular work, and it felt like my body welcomed the embryo being inserted within me, keeping it safe and healthy and able to grow. The whole process of IVF, even with donor eggs, doesn't work for some people and you're still scared you might be in that small percentage that fails, but the whole process—because of the meditation and the mind-body work—was very calming to me. I went on a lot of walks and would meditate on a lot of the things we talked about in hypnosis. I would sit on a park bench and go through the visualizations I'd learned in our sessions, about getting my family started, which is what I really wanted. It was an interesting experience, and it made my body feel very prepared.

Hypnosis was very powerful and freeing and relaxing. It helped me prepare for the pregnancy. It put me in a state that made the whole process a more beautiful than painful one. It was reassuring. I felt very confident. I used the mind-body techniques that I'd learned pre-conception throughout the pregnancy. I went full-term with my twins, who are healthy and beautiful. The doctor never put me on bed rest: my body just held these babies perfectly. I am a worrier, but I learned a lot of ways to stay positive.

One time, during the pregnancy, they thought one of my babies might have been at risk for a serious health issue. That was one of the hardest things I ever had to face: you dream about getting pregnant, then when you do, with eggs that are supposed to be fine, you could never imagine something like that going wrong. I had to wait almost two weeks for test results. I went back to my mind-body meditation work, and it helped me get through that period and regain peace of mind. Fortunately, everything turned out fine and my twins are perfectly healthy.

Having a support system like I had with a hypnotherapist, an acupuncturist, and a massage therapist, all combined to integrate things to put me in a really healthy, peaceful place to create success.

WORKS CITED

1. Christiane Northrup, *Women's Bodies, Women's Wisdom* (New York, New York: Bantam Books, 1988), 67.

2. Ibid., 209.

3. Barbara Ann Brennan, *Hands of Light* (New York, New York: Bantam Books, 1987), 127.

4. Ibid., 127.

5. Caroline Myss, *Sacred Contracts* (New York, New York: Harmony Books, 2001), 335.

6. Ibid., 165.

CHAPTER ELEVEN

THE TAO OF CONCEPTION

AN INTRODUCTION

The Tao is a five-thousand-year-old ideology that can still teach us a great deal about life and preparing for conception. It tells us that trying to use force or control or manipulation to create what we want is rarely successful because that approach is not in harmony with the laws of nature. Instead, the Tao advises us to let go of the things that have been holding us back and to find a state of inner peace within ourselves. Even in today's busy world, the most meaningful and relevant advice we receive might be the ancient wisdom and guidance of the Tao.

WHAT IS MEANT BY THE TAO

Taoism is defined in *Webster's Dictionary* as "A Chinese mystical philosophy traditionally founded by Lao-tzu in the sixth century B.C."[1] Tao translates to the word "way." It is said that Lao-tzu did not invent Taoism; instead, he simply recorded what had been a way of life in China for over two thousand years.[2] Daniel Reid, author of *The Tao of Health, Sex and Longevity*, describes the Taoist philosophy:

> Tao is a way of life, not a god or religion. It literally means "Way" or path—a trail on the journey through life which conforms to nature's own topography and time-tables.... Western ways which attempt to conquer rather than commune with the forces of nature, lead inevitably to a schizophrenic split between man and nature... To go against Tao is like trying to swim upstream against a strong

current—sooner or later you will exhaust your energy, grind to a halt, and be swept away by the cosmic currents of Tao.[3]

To live in harmony with the Tao is to be physically, mentally, and emotionally in sync with nature. This encompasses everything from nourishing our bodies with wholesome food to embracing the stillness that comes with meditation to finding a sense of peace with our past. Lao-tzu, in his immortal work, the *Tao Te Ching*, writes: "Empty yourself of everything. Let the mind rest at peace."[4] The message of the *Tao Te Ching* is that we should live our lives with unassertive action and simplicity. That means that we cannot force or control the things we want to bring into our lives, such as fertility. Instead, *the "way" or true path of manifesting what we want to create is the process of letting go, finding balance, achieving oneness with the natural world, and embracing our spirituality.* According to the Tao, everything we do that is not in harmony with nature is like swimming upstream against a strong current. In relation to fertility, it means that the *journey* is about achieving a calm state of balance that resonates with the natural world.

I am not suggesting that one needs to become a Taoist in order to conceive. Instead, I am pointing out that the principles of the Tao—letting go of old baggage, releasing the need to control or force what we want to accomplish, achieving mind-body balance, finding oneness with the universe, and opening to a higher spiritual awareness—are many of the same strategies for conception that I've been emphasizing throughout this book. In other words, the wisdom and principles of the *Tao Te Ching* are in alignment with the process of creating life, and being resistant to these five-thousand-year-old teachings might feel like moving in opposition to the flow of life.

THE TAO AND LETTING GO

Balance is achieving a state of calmness in mind, body, and spirit. One of the most important strategies in creating balance is the process of letting go and thereby creating more peace in our lives. Lao-tzu gives emphasis to this teaching when he says: "Stillness and tranquility set things in order in the universe."[5] We can only reach a state of stillness and tranquility if we let go of everything that is creating disharmony within us and release those things that are holding us back from experiencing inner peace. It is the letting go of stress and tension through meditation. It is the letting go of emotional baggage from the past that no longer serves us. It is the feeling one gets—as they do mind-body work—when they finally come to a place where they *believe* that they can overcome any obstacles that might be obstructing their path. And, it *is* about letting go of trying to control the process of becoming pregnant. One cannot be in a place of balance and, at the same time, be attempting to control aspects of their life—and their fertility. The Tao of conception is *not* about control and manipulation. It is about listening to the advice of the *Tao Te Ching* and being able to yield or let go:

> ... the ancients say, "Yield and overcome."
> Is that an empty saying?
> Be really whole,
> And all things will come to you.[6]

By yielding or letting go of all of the things that are holding us back, we can become whole or healed, and when we find that sense of harmony within us, the things we want will come to us, including pregnancy. The Tao of conception is learning how to release what is holding us back in order to reach a state of serenity where conception becomes a part of the gentle flow of nature.

THE TAO AND BALANCE

One of the primary philosophical elements of the Tao is also one of the keys to becoming pregnant: reaching a state of physical, mental, emotional, and spiritual balance. When all of those elements come to a place of harmony or inner peace, then the physical body is ready to create life. Achieving balance often means making changes that can sometimes be challenging. Acupuncturist and doctor of Oriental medicine, Angela Wu, in her book *Fertility Wisdom*, explains the importance of some of the all-encompassing changes needed to prepare for conception:

> Although you ultimately can't control the outcome of your ef-
> forts to conceive, you can do something very powerful; you can
> send an invitation by making your body a welcome place for
> new life to grow. Your physical health, your mental state, your
> emotional outlook, your lifestyle, your relationships—all send
> signals about your pregnancy readiness to the child you hope to
> attract and (even more important) carry full-term.[7]

Wu is saying that if your health, mental state, emotional outlook, lifestyle, and relationships are *out of balance*, you are *not* sending an invita-
tion to your body to get pregnant. When all opposing obstacles disappear and we achieve inner peace, our bodies become free of the
interference that can block fertility. The "way" and the fertility journey
are about balance and harmony, harmony from within and harmony
with one's *environment*.

Dr. Ted Kaptchuk, in his book about Oriental medicine, *The Web
That Has No Weaver*, explains how Chinese medicine addresses all aspects of the individual in an effort to heal the *whole* person: "The Chinese physician ... directs his or her attention to the complete physiological and psychological individual.... The therapy then attempts to bring
the configuration [the overall pattern of disharmony] into balance, to
restore harmony to the individual."[8] Harmony and balance are integral
to creating fertility. The woman who is experiencing disturbances—
whether it be stress or anger or weak kidney energy—is not in balance.
Restoring this balance through meditation, acupuncture, diet, emotional processing, lifestyle changes, and positive thought patterns helps
restore a woman to a state of harmony and inner peace.

THE TAO AND SPIRITUALITY

While spirituality is an area that is very personal for most people, and
each individual chooses their own spiritual path, it is believed that an
important aspect of balance is being in harmony with our connection
to God or Spirit or Creator or Universe, or whatever concept falls within
each person's belief system.

The philosophy of the Tao emphasizes the oneness we have with the creator of the universe as being a part of our path to enlightenment. Lao Tzu in his epic poem, *Tao Te Ching*, describes this aspect of the way as being a journey where we are moving to a place of alignment with the connection to our higher Source:

He who follows the Tao
Is at one with the Tao.
He who is virtuous
Experiences virtue.
He who loses the way
Feels lost.
When you are at one with the Tao,
The Tao welcomes you.[9]

Whereas the notion of oneness describes the connection with the universal Source; conversely, Lao-tzu points out that those individuals who are unable to be "at one with the Tao" will feel as if they have lost their way. Being in opposition or disconnected can put one in a place where they feel vulnerable and unsupported, an emptiness that is often expressed by women struggling with infertility.

Dr. Wayne Dyer, in *Real Magic,* describes how there is one universal energy that connects us all. That refers not only to being connected to our Source, but this oneness is a connection to everyone and everything in the universe:

We know there is an individual connection between all members of the human species. We know there is only one source or one energy that flows through us all. There are not millions of Gods, only one and it is in all living things, and the source of all. We call it God, yet it is called by many names. The Tao is another name given to this oneness that is in each of us.[10]

The belief that we share our energy with everything in the universe originally came from the teachings of the Buddhist religion. It was given much life by the transcendentalist movement and has now become a principle of many religions and cultures around the world.

Part of the process of manifesting a healthy body and a healthy baby may be establishing a relationship with the *Inner Source* or *Divine Power* that connects all of us. If we are in opposition or feeling disconnected or separate from our spiritual nature, that can create stress and a sense of being unsupported. However, when we are connected or in sync with universal energy, it brings the quality of inner peace into our lives and opens up the potential for us to manifest what we desire most in life.

The creation of a beautiful painting, a master work of literature, or an orchestral symphony comes initially from the Divine Source and then that brilliance is channeled into the artist, writer, or composer who gives that idea physical manifestation. Many believe that life itself is created the same way, from a Universal Source. As we build a connection with Spirit, it is that unity that gives us the ability to channel or create the things we want to manifest in our lives, including having children. Being disconnected from our Source may mean exactly that: we are separated from the energy that creates life.

For some clients on the fertility journey, the importance of this connection may be vital to their success and may be what opens the door to having a baby. Others may have no interest at all. Each person has the right to choose their own spiritual path without judgment.

It should also be noted that there is a vast difference between being *spiritual* and being *religious*. If some readers have had previous religious experiences that were negative, this does not mean they need to reconnect with that church or doctrine that felt uncomfortable in the past. Spirituality is not necessarily about following a religion. It is about one's personal relationship with God and their path of individual enlightenment. Some readers may find that their place of meditation deep within a beautiful forest becomes their *church*, and that is where they find their connection. That is perfectly acceptable, because this process is about being at peace with our connection to the oneness, which is the way of the Tao.

On this path of letting go, finding balance, achieving oneness with the natural world and embracing our spirituality we can find the insight and direction that moves us closer to fertility and enhances the quality of our lives.

In Their Own Words

Kate's story presents a striking contrast between the first part of her journey, which lasted three years and included "two surgeries, countless IVF cycles, and two failed donor cycles," and the later part where she underwent a successful IVF with donor eggs. The beginning of the journey was more about trying to force the desired outcome to materialize, whereas the last part was about achieving balance. Kate worked with meditation, visualization, and mind-body healing, all of which are natural processes. Kate also addressed the blocks that were getting in the way and was able to let go of the things that were holding her back. At the end of her story, Kate mentions how she took good care of herself with diet, acupuncture, mind-body techniques, and uterine massage. In other words, she moved into a state of mental, physical, and emotional balance much like the way of the Tao.

Kate's Story
Learning to Believe

Just a few months before getting married, my fiancé and I learned that I had numerous physical barriers to becoming pregnant. We jumped right into IVF shortly after getting married. Three years, two surgeries, countless IVF cycles, and two failed donor cycles later, we were at what appeared to be the end of the road in terms of conceiving a child. Finally, we decided to try a new donor cycle one last time with a new infertility team. Our doctor identified a new potential barrier and began treating me with an experimental medication. We were hoping that this would be our key to success. We attended a support group for couples undergoing donor cycles, as using donor ova comes with its own host of psychological and emotional issues to process.

Through this support group I met a woman who was working with several alternative reproductive therapies. This is how I came to know about hypnotherapy.

I worked with hypnosis for several months before my donor cycle was scheduled to begin. We didn't have much time, but I jumped in whole-heartedly. I wasn't sure exactly how hypnotherapy was going to help me, but I was determined to do whatever I could to make a difference in our outcome. After dealing for several years with repeated failures and disappointment, I wanted to take as much control of my situation as possible. I was tired of feeling like a victim of my own body. By undergoing hypnotherapy and practicing meditation, I learned how to visualize the inner workings of my body. I was able to visualize my infertility problems and mentally work to eradicate them. Even more importantly, I learned how to train my mind and body to do what I most wanted, to become pregnant. Every day, sometimes several times a day, I would imagine my body preparing itself for pregnancy and then becoming pregnant. I would visualize my body and all of its changes throughout the nine months of pregnancy. I would imagine the lives (as I imagined myself with twins) growing inside my womb from conception to birth.

Being able to visualize becoming pregnant and actually having babies was a very important step for me. Through all of our failed cycles, I had only come to learn and expect that I couldn't become pregnant. I had lost the ability to even imagine myself as a mother. This was an important obstacle for me to clear in order to become pregnant. On some level, I believed that it couldn't really happen. I had to retrain myself to think and believe differently. Another obstacle that I needed to address was feeling like I had to be able to endure this process alone. It was my body that had failed me, and my husband and I needed to suffer inside because of it. Hypnotherapy and meditation enabled me to identify *helpers* that I could summon at any time to help me and support me along the way. I was able to call on my own team of healers who helped to give me strength and confidence to continue forward. I had to break through my inability to accept help and support through this long and painful journey. I also had to work through the fears of what it would be like to actually become a mom and concerns about whether or not I could be a good one. I was truly uncertain if I could do a good job and if I truly deserved to be a mother. I hadn't even realized that this was an issue for me until it came up during one of the sessions. I think I spent so much energy on being infertile that I couldn't even see that there were other issues at play in my mind and body.

After going through this final donor cycle, we became pregnant with twins. I continued with my daily meditation and visualization throughout my pregnancy. I had healthy full-term babies—a boy and a girl. I am grateful to our medical team as I believe that the experimental medication helped me to become pregnant, but I am also confident that all of the mind-body work that I did also played a significant role in our success. I truly believe that I was open to becoming pregnant and ready to become a good mother as a result of all of my work. I visualized the entire process, from the effectiveness of the medication through the births of my healthy twins. My mind helped my body to perform as I needed it to. I took such good care of myself. I sought the help of acupuncture, I changed my diet and I received uterine massage. I did everything in my power to become pregnant, more than in any other stage of my infertility journey. I felt very empowered by doing so. Finally, I had taken the power and control back.

I know that I found hope and strength through the mind-body connection. I feel like almost anything can be possible when you choose to truly believe.

WORKS CITED

1. *Webster's Seventh New Collegiate Dictionary* (Springfield, Massachusetts: G. C. Merriam Company, 1967), 901.

2. Daniel Reid, *The Tao of Health, Sex and Longevity* (New York, New York: Fireside Books, 1989), 3.

3. Ibid., 3.

4. Gia-Fu Feng, and Jane English (translators). Original text by Lao Tsu. *Tao Te Ching* (New York, New York: Vintage Books, 1972), Verse 16.

5. Ibid., Verse 45.

6. Ibid., Verse 22.

7. Angela Wu, *Fertility Wisdom* (Emmaus, PA: Rodale Books, 2006), 51.

8. Ted Kaptchuk, *The Web That Has No Weaver* (New York, New York: Congdon & Weed, 1983), 4.

9. Feng, "Tao-te Ching," Verse 23.

10. Wayne Dyer, *Real Magic* (New York, New York: Harper Collins Books, 1992), 125–6.

CHAPTER TWELVE

PREPARING FOR CONCEPTION:
A Timeline and Action Plan

How does one begin the journey of becoming pregnant? Are there steps, such as lifestyle changes, that can be beneficial? At what point does one seek assistance? What options are available in medical reproductive technology, and what are the alternative or complementary modalities? What are the tools and techniques that can make this a journey of self-discovery and empowerment rather than a long period of difficulty, frustration, and despair?

In this chapter, I provide an action plan to help guide women through the process of getting their minds and bodies ready to conceive, including information about alternative therapies and traditional treatments so that women know what steps to take to maximize their chances of becoming pregnant. These recommendations—which are not a substitute for medical advice—are based on a great deal of research, input from experts who work in this field, and experience and observations I have made in my work with infertility. Finally, I have included a self-test so that women can see if there are areas where they can improve their potential for conception.

Since some readers, in their eagerness to move forward, are going to read this chapter first, I've briefly summarized *some* of the information presented throughout the book. However, knowledge is true empowerment, and to get a clear understanding of the concepts, it is important to go back and find out why certain approaches to fertility are so much more effective than others.

ACTION PLAN:
THE FIRST SIX TO TWELVE MONTHS

Step 1: Reduce Stress

A. Start Practicing a Daily Meditation

Nothing in this journey is more important than stress reduction. If the body and mind are not calm, it is almost impossible for conception to take place. As discussed earlier in this book, when a woman is experiencing stress, it adversely affects the mind's control center for reproductive activity, the hypothalamus gland. Tension and anxiety cause the body to react by switching *on* the sympathetic nervous system, which puts the body into the survival—*not the reproductive*—mode. When this dynamic is created, it essentially turns *off* the body's ability to become pregnant. In plain and simple terms, a woman who is experiencing physical, mental, or emotional stress is unplugging her ability to conceive.

Are there exceptions? Yes, but they are becoming increasingly rare. A woman who is stressed at age twenty-one may still be able to conceive because her body is young and strong and she is in her peak fertility years. A woman who is anxious might be able to override her body's off switch and get pregnant after numerous IVF procedures—and perhaps the use of donor eggs—but even one IVF procedure is taxing on both the body and the pocketbook. Women who attempt to circumvent doing stress reduction work by using in vitro procedures will often spend tens of thousands of dollars and still end up without a baby. So, for women who aren't twenty-one and women who don't have unlimited financial resources, the essential starting point in the fertility journey is to reduce stress. If stress isn't addressed, it is very doubtful that any time and money spent on traditional Western or even alternative methods to promote pregnancy will produce positive results. *It all begins with stress management.*

Stress reduction should become part of a daily routine. An activity such as meditation should be practiced each morning in order to promote a feeling of peace within the body and to establish the intention— what one wishes to create—for the day. Meditation is best learned from an individual teacher or by taking a class. If this is not possible, working daily with an audio recording of a stress reduction or fertility meditation can be beneficial in quieting the mind.

B. Address the Origins of Stress

Use a technique such as hypnotherapy to identify and process emotional issues that are generating stress in your life and creating blocks to your fertility. As I discussed in chapter three, stress is the direct result of our emotional issues, and those issues are commonly overlooked because the word "stress" has become associated *only* with our daily routines. *This is a serious misconception because oftentimes people experiencing stress will simply examine their day-to-day schedule and disregard the real source of what is impacting their fertility.* It is true that the day-to-day stuff will often need to be addressed, but that usually makes up only a small part of the overall stress picture that is affecting our bodies and blocking conception. *The majority of the stress is coming from our unprocessed issues, past and present.*

The person who says, "I've already worked on all my stuff," will almost always find that there are deeper levels or other aspects of the material they have already explored that are revealed as soon as they access their subconscious mind. "I've already worked on all my stuff," is often a statement of denial. Having a willingness to look within opens the path to enlightenment.

The most important step in stress reduction is identifying and healing whatever baggage we have that is directly connected to infertility. Of all the steps on this list, processing the old issues is probably the most important, because those old issues are creating the majority of the stress that we feel. The day-to-day stuff may compound those uncomfortable feelings in the body, but the roots of that discomfort come from our past. Hypnotherapy is the best tool to accomplish this because in order to be successful in this work, one has to deal directly with the material in the subconscious mind. This is not a procedure that can be carried out with the conscious mind.

C. Disconnect the Present-Day Stress that Drains Your Energy

Sometimes it is easier to understand the concept of how our issues and subsequent stress can affect us by thinking of our bodies as running on or being fueled by energy. Naturally, a focus on energy flow is the basis for Eastern medicine, but on an even simpler level, everyone understands the basics of feeling *energized, inspired,* or *joyful* as opposed to what it feels like when we feel *drained, exhausted* or *defeated.*

Our issues—past and present—can drain our energy. For example, a woman who is unhappy with her job or puts in lots of overtime might feel drained when she gets home because she is giving away all of her energy at the workplace. Sometimes a family member such as a meddling in-law or irresponsible sibling might become an energy drain. Even situations like unsettled living conditions such as residing in a noisy apartment or a house undergoing a remodeling project can be exhausting. These are just a few examples of present-day issues that can take away vital energy that the body needs for reproduction.

Most women reading this book are in their thirties and forties and, unlike women in their early twenties, they need *all* of their energy to create a healthy conception. A woman who works fifty to sixty hours a week may leave herself with only 30 percent of her energy to keep her reproductive organs nurtured and strong. A couple who is experiencing financial difficulties may be giving 60 percent of their energy to concerns about how to get out of debt. A woman who has experienced a miscarriage may be losing 50 percent of her energy to fears that she might miscarry again. Those numbers might reflect what we give away to individual issues, but realistically, we all have numerous issues in our lives that create our stress. *Many women who want to get pregnant are giving away the very energy that they need for successful reproduction to take place.*

Make an honest evaluation of your present situation. If your body is exhausted or if the mind is consumed with worry or frustration over things like how much you dislike your job or present-day conflicts with people in your life or other extraneous situations, you are probably giving away the energy needed to get pregnant. A promise to cut back on the workload or address the issues "as soon as I am pregnant" is simply leaving the conception switch in the off position and hoping for a miracle. The physical body requires rest and inner peace in order to perform all of the functions—such as producing viable follicles—for conception to take place.

Step 2: Eliminate Tobacco and Alcohol

There isn't much need to explain why this is important because there is so much medical research to support taking these steps.

Many women ask if they can just have a glass or two of wine a week during this process. Dr. Mark Leondires, an expert on reproductive medicine, says that alcohol—even in moderate drinkers—can disrupt the ovulatory and menstrual cycles in women. He goes on to say that the depressant effect of alcohol can also affect sperm production.[1] So, the best advice for those who want to maximize their chances of becoming pregnant is to eliminate alcohol altogether.

There have been numerous studies about the impact tobacco has on the body's ability to conceive. This is not a negotiable issue: a woman shouldn't even begin the process of trying to conceive until she is tobacco-free. The physiological impact on the mother's body is extremely detrimental to the conception process, and, if one does get pregnant, it presents a very unhealthy situation for the developing embryo.

Many women who want to get pregnant but fail to give up tobacco are unable to conceive because of the guilt factor; they know how smoking can affect the health of a child, and the subconscious mind sends unfavorable messages to the body, thereby blocking the body's ability to conceive.

In regard to the most effective method for eliminating tobacco, a study conducted at Texas A & M in 2004, where hypnosis was used for smoking cessation, found that 81 percent of the subjects using this method were able to stop smoking.[2] Another study, conducted at the University of Washington, which also utilized hypnosis for smoking cessation posted a 90.6 percent success rate.[3] The long-term success rate for the patch is 7–9 percent and nicotine gum is less than 5 percent.[4]

Step 3: Eliminate Coffee, Caffeine, Soft Drinks and Artificial Sweeteners

According to Dr. Leondires, "even one cup of coffee per day can reduce a woman's chances of getting pregnant within a twelve-month period by more than 50 percent." Leondires goes on to say that three cups a day will drop the odds by more than 175 percent.[5] Caffeine has an addictive effect on the body and weakens the adrenal glands, over time, by over-stimulating them. The adrenal glands communicate with the hypothalamus gland; excessive stimulation sends a signal that the body is in stress mode. If a person feels addiction withdrawal when stopping coffee (headaches, extreme fatigue, and irritability), then they can be helped with acupuncture and herbs that replenish and repair the adrenal glands.

Many women might think they can simply switch to soft drinks, but it is widely believed that caffeine (an ingredient in many soft drinks) and the sweeteners used in these types of beverages are all culprits when it comes to interfering with fertility. Soft drinks are either sweetened by sugar, which interferes with normal glucose levels in the blood and can lead to diabetes, or artificial sweeteners. Artificial sweeteners have become very popular in our society because so many products are marketed as sugar-free. One of the most common artificial sweeteners is aspartame which, according to health and fitness expert Noah Hittner, "... breaks down into wood-alcohol (methanol), which is essentially embalming fluid."[6] Hittner says aspartame has the potential to "[aggravate] diabetes mellitus, [and contribute to] hypoglycemia, convulsions, headache, depression, other psychiatric states, hyperthyroidism, hypertension, arthritis, the simulation of multiple sclerosis, Alzheimer's disease, lupus erythematosus, carpal tunnel syndrome—to name only a few."[7] The other commonly used sweetener, Splenda or sucralose, according to Hittner, is a combination of sugar and chlorine "known for causing organ, genetic, and reproductive damage."[8] Whether or not one is interested in conceiving, these sweeteners should be eliminated from the diet. Healthier substitutes include the herb stevia and xylatol, a natural product that comes from the bark of birch trees. Good beverage choices for women trying to conceive include decaffeinated green tea, herbal teas, 100-percent natural fruit drinks (without corn syrup), and natural spring water. Some dark, full-bodied teas make good substitutes for coffee. These healthy beverage and sugar substitutes can be purchased at health food stores.

Step 4: Focus on a Healthy Diet

What we put into our bodies provides fuel and helps us create healthy chi or energy. The food we eat converts into energy that supports all of the life functions within our bodies. If we want our bodies to perform at optimum levels, then we need to nourish ourselves with healthy meals. When the fuel we put into our bodies isn't comprised of nutritious food, then our bodies can fail to function to their maximum potential. In regard to fertility, people with healthy eating habits are enhancing their chances of a successful pregnancy.

Many foods on the market today do not nourish our physical bodies. For example, foods that are high in sugar and/or white flour have little nutritious value, and, as a result, provide little or no fuel to support life functions. Foods that are high in salt or unhealthy fats can make us feel sluggish or heavy, and affect our bodies and our health in an adverse way. Foods that are high in chemicals, such as artificial sweeteners, coloring agents, or preservatives, can introduce toxins into our system. Meats and dairy products that have been stimulated by hormones may be introducing unnatural synthetic chemicals into our body's delicate hormonal balance.

The best guideline for eating-to-conceive is to eat fresh, organic foods. Organic fruits and vegetables—especially the brightly colored ones such as broccoli, green beans, spinach, carrots, squash, blueberries, apples, peaches, and apricots—should become a staple in the diet of anyone wanting to conceive. Experts recommend five portions a day, and that is a great way to nurture your body.

Foods that are not organic often contain toxic chemicals. These unnatural agents, when introduced into our bodies, interfere with our ability to function at our full potential. It has been well documented that pesticides have created infertility in numerous animal species. Is it safe to assume that we are immune to these chemical toxins? We may not know, at this time, the full extent of how things such as pesticides, preservatives, artificial hormones, saturated fats, coloring agents, and sweeteners affect the functions within our bodies, but common sense tells us that it cannot be good for us. Organic products are available in almost all grocery stores and are prevalent in health food stores. These products are finally available and affordable to the masses because there is a strong demand from health-conscious consumers. I recommend that everyone eat fresh, organic foods, especially women who want to get pregnant.

Consuming high amounts of refined carbohydrates such as products made from white flour can not only lead to serious health issues (such as obesity and diabetes), but these substances fail to provide adequate nutrients and energy to support reproductive functions. It should be noted that many reproductive experts, including Dr. Randine Lewis and Dr. Angela Wu, recommend that women who want to get pregnant should eliminate all wheat- and gluten-containing grains from their diets. The number of people who experience various levels of wheat and/or gluten intolerance in our society is beginning to reach disturbing levels. In many cases, this type of intolerance is overlooked until the symptoms it creates become more extreme. One reason for this is that this type of intolerance will not always show up in standard blood tests. The other reason is that gluten intolerances can vary in degree of severity and in symptomology. Milder cases can include symptoms such as skin rashes, headaches, chronic bloating, candida overgrowth, bone and joint pain, and general fatigue. In many instances, people will fail to associate these symptoms with the consumption of wheat and/or gluten. More serious wheat and gluten reactions can include severe bloating, digestive distress, and irritable bowel conditions. Some experts believe that wheat and gluten intolerance may be a factor in infertility.

Consumption of dairy products by women wishing to conceive should be minimal and those products should always be organic and free of hormones. From an Eastern medicine perspective, the intake of dairy creates a damp stagnation condition in the uterus. This makes the uterus an unfavorable environment for implantation. If calcium intake is a concern, focus on consuming large amounts of dark, green vegetables and consider taking a good quality calcium supplement. Doctors recommend a good prenatal vitamin/mineral combination to be taken before conception to provide adequate folic acid and other essential nutrients. Some calcium will be provided in this pre-natal supplement, but it may still not be adequate.

Holistic experts caution that cold raw foods, iced beverages, and frozen desserts should be avoided. This is because they create a chill inside the body. The body should be kept more like a warm nest for easy conception. Even fresh vegetables should be lightly steamed, and salads should be consumed with warm tea or soup to neutralize their intrinsic cooling nature.

The protein we eat forms the building blocks for many of our life processes and helps regulate our blood sugar for sustained energy. The quality of the protein consumed is an important consideration. Organic poultry, beef, and mercury-free fish are good choices. I suggest that women consume some protein—either animal or vegetable based—at each of their meals. This can sometimes be a challenge for women who are vegetarians, as they may need to pay special attention to food combining to make sure they are getting complete proteins. Vegetarians should also consult the latest research on the over-consumption of soy and the negative effect that may have on the thyroid gland.

Harvard researchers compiling information from 18,000 women who took part in the Nurses Health Study made several recommendations about diet and its effects on fertility. They report that eating "easily digested carbohydrates (fast carbs) such as white bread, potatoes, and sugared sodas increases the odds that you'll find yourself struggling with ovulatory infertility."[9] Conversely, they found that eating slowly digested carbohydrates that are high in fiber will improve fertility. It was no surprise that the study found that trans fats increase infertility. Their recommendation was that women should eat a limited amount of healthful unsaturated fats, and found that women who eat too little fat often struggle with conception.[10] In regard to protein, the study recommends that "getting more protein from plants and less from animals is another big step toward walking away from infertility."[11]

It goes without saying that fast food and junk food should be eliminated completely. These foods have a high content of salt, fats, processed carbohydrates, and sugars, all of which throw the body into metabolic imbalance.

A healthy diet forms the basis of a healthy life, strengthening the immune system and promoting vitality. Following the guidelines above—which are based on recommendations by experts in this field—can not only make you feel better, but can also prepare your body for conception.

Step 5: Implement an Appropriate Exercise Program

The most commonly recommended exercise for women wanting to enhance their fertility is yoga. Yoga is a form of exercise that focuses on stretching, strengthening, and relaxing the body. It is also known for its ability to reduce stress without physically taxing the body, unlike many aerobic exercises. There are various forms of yoga and this recommendation is specifically for the types of yoga that emphasize gentle movement and quieting the mind. A woman who wants to get pregnant should *avoid* doing any form of hot, extreme, or bikram yoga because these forms create too much stress on the physical body.

Other physical activities beneficial for promoting conception that are good for moving energy and quieting the mind are Tai Chi and Qi Gong.

Walking, swimming, and moderate bike riding are also good activities that provide exercise and are complementary to the conception process.

Experts now suggest that we get thirty to forty minutes of cardiovascular work four to five times a week. Women who are exceeding this are putting their bodies under too much physical stress, releasing too much adrenaline, and they are giving away the physical energy their bodies need to reproduce.

I talked earlier in this chapter about giving away energy to stressors, such as dysfunctional job situations, and how that can drain one's life force, but another way that many women give up their physical energy is by excessive exercising. This is especially common for women who are overly concerned with body image and/or women who fall into the perfectionist category (described in chapter seven). According to Dr. Ronald Wilbois, medical director of the infertility and IVF center in St. Louis, over-exercising can lead to ovulatory dysfunction. Wilbois also says that excessive exercise will cause the body to produce adrenaline "which is interpreted by the body as stress."[12] Our bodies can't distinguish between stress from excessive exercise and stress from life-threatening situations. As a result, the hypothalamus gland, sensing being overwhelmed from too much exercise, sends a signal to the body to enter fight-or-flight, or survival mode, thus moving the body out of conception mode. All of these physiological responses are explained in chapter four, but the key point is that too much exercise or exercise that is too extreme can cause the physical body to decrease proper reproductive functioning.

Runners are a good example of this. They are, often, greatly reducing their ability to conceive by expending energy that the body needs for healthy reproductive functioning. They are depleting their reproductive life force, which is known as kidney energy in Chinese medicine. Running creates a stress response in the hypothalamus gland (described above and in chapter four) and triggers the release of adrenaline produced by the adrenal glands. Runners say that this activity relaxes them, but paradoxically the "adrenaline high" is really a form of physical stress as the body is in fight-or-flight mode.

Another serious consequence of running is the cumulative effect of the pounding motion on the uterus, an organ held in place by stretchable ligaments. The bouncing or pounding from running or jogging is a common cause of uterine misalignment. When the uterus is out of alignment (tilted forward, backward, or sideways), it can cause several conditions that are detrimental to fertility: the reproductive pathway can become seriously occluded or closed off, the lymph drainage system may not be able to properly eliminate old waste material that needs to be removed from the body, and, most importantly, the menstrual blood collected monthly in the uterus may not drain properly. An indication of blood that is pooling or not fully draining from the uterus is menstrual blood that is *not* bright red. If there is a brownish color or clotting quality to this blood, it often indicates the blood in the uterus is old blood and it is likely that the uterus may be out of its proper position. If the uterus is partially filled with old blood that hasn't been draining properly, that means an embryo isn't receiving the rich, nutritious blood it needs to grow and develop. Fortunately, this can be corrected with Maya uterine massage (discussed in greater detail in chapter thirteen).

Another issue for runners, centering around the pounding effect on the uterus, is whether a newly fertilized embryo would have the ability to implant and to stay in place inside a uterus that is being subjected to jostling or bouncing on a regular basis.

Women who want to conceive need to stop running. For some, this is hard. I've observed women change practitioners who've given them this advice—rather than stop running—when they are told to do so. A woman can choose between getting pregnant or continuing to be a runner. More often than not, she can't have it both ways.

Women who have been active athletes for many years often have an identity of themselves as vigorous women who are able to compete and excel in physical activities. This is no longer appropriate when the objective is to promote conception. Bursts of exercise that were once invigorating may now be depleting the physical body. Running can always be resumed after a woman has achieved her goal and fully recovered from the birthing process.

Step 6: Take an Honest Look at Your Weight

Some women may need to address weight concerns. Fertility can be an issue for both over- and underweight women. The Nurses Health Study, compiled by researchers at Harvard University, had this to say about body weight: "Weighing too much or weighing too little can interrupt normal menstrual cycles, throw off ovulation or stop it altogether."[13]

Many studies have shown that women who are significantly overweight have difficulty becoming pregnant. They may have insulin resistance, a condition where "too much insulin circulates in the body, disrupting menstruation."[14] Another issue for women who are overweight is that "estrogen production from fat cells can also affect the ovaries and prevent eggs from being released every month—a condition called *anovulation.*"[15] Many women in this situation mistakenly believe they are consistently ovulating because they have regular periods, but this is not necessarily true.

Woman who are underweight also have difficulty with conception and carrying full term. According to Dr. Helen Kim, assistant professor of obstetrics and gynecology, and director of the in vitro fertilization program at the University of Chicago, women who are underweight, with a low body mass index, take "four times as long to get pregnant as women in the normal range."[16]

Being five to ten pounds overweight is *not* a problem for women trying to conceive; however, five or more pounds underweight *does* seem to make the process more difficult.

Women who are underweight often tend to over-exercise, eat small quantities of food, skip meals, eat on the run, and consume too many fast-burning carbohydrates and not enough protein. Again, protein is essential to keep our energy steady and regulate blood sugar levels. These lifestyle habits create imbalances that cause deficiencies in the body and can make it unable to reproduce.

The best way to honestly evaluate your weight is to consult a height vs. body weight chart or take a body mass index test, and take appropriate action based on what the *experts* feel is the proper weight for you. This should not be based on your opinion, as our own personal weight assessments are often inaccurate.

Step 7: Experience Acupuncture

Acupuncture (described in more detail in chapter 13) is designed to create balance in the body. A practitioner of Eastern medicine works with the energy—also called life force or chi—in the body to create that balance. Energy within our bodies flows along what are called meridians or energy pathways. When the energy flows evenly through the meridians to all of our organs, it creates balance within the body. If energy within a meridian system or an internal organ is imbalanced, that can create disharmony in the body. Again, energy is the key, and acupuncture is a means of balancing that energy to nourish the reproductive system.

From the Eastern medicine perspective, most individuals, when they reach their thirties, start to experience a drop-off in the energy or chi within the kidneys. This doesn't mean that anything is wrong with them, it is simply a fact that over the course of one's life, the kidneys are unable

to produce energy at the same levels that they were able to maintain decades earlier. The kidney energy, according to Eastern medicine, is what
generates the life force in the reproductive system. When an acupuncturist observes that the energy coming from the kidneys is depleted, they
use acupuncture and herbs to strengthen the kidneys, which, in turn, creates a healthy energy flow to the reproductive organs.

While this is a very simplified example of how acupuncture can
treat infertility—and only a very small piece of the true complexities
addressed by an Eastern medicine practitioner when they treat infertility—it is included here to point out how energy deficiencies at the root
of infertility can often be successfully treated with acupuncture. Correcting the root of the problem may—for many women—circumvent
the need for Western medical interventions.

I recommend that a woman work with an acupuncturist for at least
six months at the beginning of her fertility journey. Eastern medicine
looks at infertility in a very different way than Western medicine. The
focus of the acupuncturist is on correcting imbalances and energy disruptions in the body by looking at the root or source of these issues.
Many women find that once they have established a healthy energetic
balance in their body, they are able to conceive on their own.

Many acupuncturists are also licensed to work with herbs. Using
herbs can greatly enhance a woman's progress and success rate in this
work, but it should be noted that it is not recommended to combine
herbs with some of the Western medical drugs used to promote conception. It is best to consult your doctor about that matter.

I firmly believe that acupuncture and hypnosis are two synergistic
modalities that are not only complementary to one another, but work
in these modalities can potentiate or make stronger the work that can
be done by using either modality on its own. A hypnotist familiar with
Eastern medicine and mind-body healing can incorporate the Eastern
medicine strategies into a personalized meditation for his or her clients
with very powerful results.

Step 8: Schedule a Maya Uterine Massage

Maya uterine massage is described in greater detail in chapter thirteen. I also explain why this process is recommended in the exercise section in this chapter. While runners and former athletes often have problems with misplacement issues concerning the uterus, this can also happen with women who have been in car accidents, have done a great deal of heavy lifting, have had a baby or miscarriage, or have experienced any one of a number of other conditions.

The objective of this work is to make sure that the uterus is in proper alignment in order for pregnancy to occur. Most practitioners who do Maya uterine massage need to see a client at least twice. The practitioner will teach the client how to do daily self-massage exercises to maintain the proper positioning of her uterus. I believe that if the uterus is out of alignment, it can greatly reduce one's chances of becoming pregnant.

Summary

I have found that many women following the above steps can successfully conceive within twelve months. Holistic modalities and lifestyle changes are a bridge to natural conception. In the process of following these steps, most women report increased vitality, an improved state of physical and emotional well-being, and they are motivated to make many of these practices lifetime habits.

In my opinion, if after all of the holistic modalities have been utilized, and pregnancy still has not occurred after twelve months, then a woman may choose to pursue assisted reproductive technologies. It is still advisable to complement Western medical strategies with holistic techniques so that a balanced mind and body is in place before undergoing any medical procedures.

Assisted reproductive technology is constantly changing, so the information presented here is simply intended to provide a general idea of some of the steps a woman can take if she chooses to utilize Western medicine. To get the most up-to-date and accurate information on Western medical procedures, a woman should consult her doctor.

ACTION PLAN:

MONTHS TWELVE THROUGH TWENTY-FOUR

Continue Following Steps 1–8 Listed Above

Step 9: Schedule The Medical Workup

Infertility is defined as the inability to achieve a pregnancy after twelve months of unprotected intercourse. After trying to conceive for a year and taking advantage of the modalities listed above, it is recommended that a patient see her obstetrician/gynecologist (OB/GYN) for an evaluation. The OB/GYN can determine if more extensive tests are needed, at which time a referral will be made to a reproductive endocrinologist (a medical fertility specialist). Blood work and a series of tests to check hormone levels, blocked fallopian tubes, endometriosis, etc., will be conducted to ascertain if there are physical issues that need to be addressed. Both the male and female should be tested because approximately 30–40 percent of infertility can be due to male factor infertility.

The Medical Workup

Although the medical workup itself is necessary, what happens after that evaluation can often be disconcerting. Once this step is taken, it usually plunges couples directly into the Western medical protocols with little or no regard to complementary modalities. Couples are often advised about their next steps strictly in the context of Western medicine. These medical recommendations are often associated with inferences such as "you'd better act now before it's too late," or "given your age, you have no other choice," which creates added pressure, clouds the decision-making process, and establishes a mindset that this is the *only* solution.

An example of this is the follicle-stimulating hormone (FSH) test. When a woman goes in for a medical evaluation, she is given an FSH test to evaluate ovarian function, which many experts use as an indicator of her ability to conceive. For many women, the results of this test can make or break their world. The common assumption—an assumption with which many holistic practitioners disagree—is that a high FSH test means that a woman's life-long dream of having her own biological children is not a possibility. If a woman's FSH is high, she might be advised to undergo an in vitro procedure with donor eggs. However, it is extremely important to put this all in context. FSH is a hormone: a follicle stimulating hormone. Hormones are controlled by the hypothalamus gland. As I have documented many times in this book, the hypothalamus gland is highly susceptible to stress and that, in turn, affects the regulation of hormones in the body. A woman who hasn't conceived for a year is already very stressed—doing a battery of tests that may indicate that she is unable to have a baby can generate monumental levels of anxiety. Under these circumstances, is it likely that a woman's FSH will fall into the normal range? The medical community has scientific research to document that stress has a *very* significant effect on the hypothalamus gland and the production of hormones. Are we supposed to believe that the hormones related to reproductive activity are the *one and only exception*, the only hormones in the body that are not influenced by stress? That is extremely unlikely. After years of experience in working with infertility clients, Dr. Elizabeth Muir says: "In my opinion, FSH level is very much affected by the level of stress...."[17] Thus, an elevated FSH score, created by high stress levels, may lead a woman to believe donor eggs and an in vitro procedure are her *only* choice when, in fact, there are several other factors to be considered.

Furthermore, we have to look at the significance of the *power of suggestion* (discussed in chapter six) in these situations. The power of suggestion—where an idea, concept, or fear is introduced into one's belief system—is greatly magnified when it is introduced under two specific conditions: during a stressful situation or when it is delivered by a person of authority. If the new information comes at a time when we are stressed or in despair, such as when undergoing a critical infertility examination, it can be especially potent. The other factor that can enhance that power of suggestion is when the prognosis comes from a person of authority, such as a doctor. In this context, both of these conditions are in full force, often resulting in a singular belief about how to best approach the infertile situation. Whatever words are spoken at that time can instantly become the law that governs all thought and action.

I've had many women, who were in that situation, tell me that they had such a strong emotional reaction after the doctor said the words "high FSH" that they can't remember a thing their doctor said after that diagnosis. Due to the power of suggestion, a negative diagnosis can instantly become a part of that woman's belief system. Women will leave the doctor's office *believing* that they have no other choice but to pursue the Western medical strategies. And, for some women, Western medicine might be a good choice. However, there are many pathways to fertility, and it is important to not get overwhelmed by powerful statements that cause us to feel a sense of urgency and pressure to succumb to procedures based on one opinion and our subsequent emotions.

It is important to remember that a woman and her partner, at the time of the medical evaluation, are in a highly suggestible state. It doesn't mean that the information should be disregarded; it simply means that it is only *one measure* of their fertility. It is one opinion based on a test that may be skewed because of the stress element. All options should be carefully weighed and explored before making any rash decisions. Sometimes the pressure that a woman and her partner feel is likely to push them into the Western medical program, without their even considering working with alternatives or addressing issues such as the stress that might be creating the true dynamics of the situation. If a woman has spent a year working with holistic modalities, then it may be time to consider the Western medical approach; however, many women choose the Western medical approach first without preparing their minds and bodies by using holistic modalities.

So, while the workup is necessary to check for physical issues, it can often create a situation where other options are overlooked and couples feel pressured to solely pursue Western medical channels. Furthermore, if some of the issues, such as the stress factor, are not under control, it is unlikely that pregnancy will occur, with or without assisted reproductive techniques.

In conclusion, the Western medical workup is advisable, but it is important to be open-minded, take a balanced approach, and make use of all tools and modalities available.

Step 10: Stimulation Drugs and Intrauterine Insemination (IUI)

If the results of the fertility exam indicate that there are no significant medical issues preventing conception, the patient will often start the Western medical process with an intrauterine insemination (IUI). An IUI consists of hormone treatments to stimulate follicle production and then a series of ultrasounds to make sure follicles (not cysts) are being produced. When the woman is ovulating, she and her husband go into the doctor's office. The husband donates sperm, which is washed and then injected through a flexible catheter directly into the uterus through the cervix. Same-sex couples, single mothers, and couples experiencing male factor infertility can use donated sperm to take advantage of this process. The cost for this procedure, including the stimulation drugs, is usually about $1,500 to $3,000. This procedure will often be attempted three to four times. The success rate for this procedure is typically 2–8 percent, although some studies claim higher numbers with multiple follicles, injectable medications, etc.

Male factor infertility, which includes low sperm counts, poor sperm motility (ability to swim), or issues with sperm morphology (distorted shapes of the sperm) can be the cause of infertility in about 25 percent of the cases, and a contributing factor 30–40 percent of the time. The Western medical approach to sperm issues can include techniques such as interuterine inseminations, in vitro procedures with ICSI (intra-cytoplasmic sperm injection, where the sperm is injected directly into the egg), or sperm donation. However, if the male works with an acupuncturist and takes herbs, many sperm issues can show dramatic improvement. It is important to note that the sperm released today is produced ninety days prior to its release. Therefore, working with an acupuncturist—often on a once-a-week basis—should occur for a period of at least ninety days in order to generate effective results.

Step 11: In Vitro Fertilization (IVF)

If the attempts with intrauterine insemination IUIs are unsuccessful, the next step is to undergo in vitro fertilization (IVF). Some women will bypass the IUIs if they are older or using donor eggs. The first step is to stimulate the production of follicles through the use of stimulation drugs. The second step, called the retrieval, is when the doctor goes in and removes the stimulated follicles to be used for the procedure. The follicles are united with the sperm in vitro, meaning "in the laboratory." The final step is the transfer. This is the part of the procedure where the fertilized eggs are put back into the woman's uterus. Same sex couples, single mothers, and couples where there is male factor infertility may choose in vitro fertilization if they have not found success with intra-uterine insemination. The cost for an IVF runs approximately $12,000 to $25,000. The success rate for all IVFs is approximately 28 percent, according to the ART report issued by the CDC, although the numbers can vary widely, depending on the age of the woman, the use of adjunct procedures such ICSI, and the use of donor eggs (see chapter two for a more detailed explanation).

FERTILITY SELF-TEST

Are there areas where you could improve your ability to conceive? This test is a self-evaluation to see if there are things you could do to enhance your fertility. Enter your answers in the left-hand column. Enter only one number for each blank. Choose the number that best applies to your situation. You can enter a zero or leave a blank space for those issues that don't apply to you.

Begin with Your Positive Habits

_____ If you have read this book, give yourself 100 points to start the quiz.

_____ If you are receiving acupuncture, add 15 points to your score.

_____ If you have been receiving acupuncture for at least 3–6 months, you can instead add 25 points to your score.

_____ If you are using the daily self-massage techniques of Maya uterine massage to make sure that your uterus is in proper alignment, add 20 points.

_____ If you have done hypnotherapy or any kind of therapy that directly addresses the *subconscious* issues, add 25 points to your score.

_____ If you are doing a daily meditation with visualization, you can add 20 points to your score.

Subtract the Negative Habits

_____ If you drink more than 2–3 alcoholic drinks a week, subtract 10 points; more than 4–5 alcoholic drinks a week, subtract 25 points.

_____ If you drink coffee or a caffeinated drink every day, subtract 25 points.

_____ If you drink more than two soft drinks a week, subtract 15 points; more than five soft drinks a week, subtract 25 points.

_____ If you eat fast food more than once a week, subtract 10 points; more than three times a week, subtract 25 points.

_____ If you eat junk food more than three times a week, subtract 10 points; more than five times a week, subtract 25 points.

_____ If your diet contains preservatives, hormones, coloring agents or other chemical additives more than three times a week, subtract 10 points; more than five times a week, subtract 20 points.

_____ If your diet contains artificial sweeteners more than once a week, subtract 10 points; more than three times a week, subtract 25 points.

_____ If you eat sweets/desserts/candy more than three times a week, subtract 10 points; more than five times a week, subtract 25 points.

_____ If you eat foods made with white processed flour more than three times a week, subtract 10 points; more than five times a week, subtract 25 points.

_____ If you exercise (with the exception of calming meditative yoga) more than 5 hours a week, subtract 10 points; more than 8 hours a week, subtract 25 points.

_____ If you are a runner, subtract 25 points.

_____ If you exercise once a week or not at all, subtract 20 points.

_____ If you are extremely unhappy or extremely stressed with your work situation, subtract 25 points.

_____ If you work over 40 hours a week, subtract 10 points; more than 50 hours a week, subtract 25 points; 60 or more hours a week, subtract 50 points.

_____ If you have a day-to-day situation, outside of work, that is an energy drain (such as a difficult family member), subtract 25 points.

_____ If you are more than 40 pounds overweight, subtract 25 points; 20–39 pound overweight, subtract 15 points.

_____ If, according to medical charts, your body weight is five to ten pounds under what is considered normal for your height, subtract 15 points; more than ten pounds under, subtract 25 points.

_____ If you have never done any processing of your issues, but know you have "baggage," subtract 25 points.

_____ If you smoke, subtract 100 points.

_____ Total

While the numbers assigned here are not scientific, the objective is to assist you in determining how many factors may be standing in the way of your pregnancy. Your score in this self-test may not be as important as taking a look at the areas where you could be doing more to maximize your chances of getting pregnant. Any item that generated a score of 25 should be considered an area that needs to be addressed.

Keep in mind that this test is not intended to promote a compulsive response where you try to do everything perfectly. Perfection, as discussed in chapter seven, is one of the biggest blocks to conception. The goal is to practice moderation. For example, the woman who has one piece of chocolate every night after dinner or one or two small desserts a week is probably not going to hurt her chances of getting pregnant. Conversely, the woman who always has a candy bar at the office and a big bowl of ice cream for dessert every night, might be hurting her ability to conceive. I suggest that women simply use this self-test as a guide and change habits to achieve moderation, *not perfection.*

TEST RESULTS

If your score is:

190–90: Excellent. You are already doing a lot of beneficial work to enhance your fertility.

89–70: Good. You are doing well overall, but there is potential to boost your chances of conceiving.

69–50: Average. There may be areas that need attention to improve your situation.

49 and below: Poor. There are several areas that need to be addressed, but now you know what needs to be changed to begin your journey.

WORKS CITED

1. Mark Leondires, "Are Your Vices Preventing You From Becoming Pregnant?" *Achieving Families*, www.achievingfamilies.com, 12.

2. G. R. Elkins and M. H. Rajab, "Clinical hypnosis for smoking cessation: preliminary results of a three-session intervention" Texas A&M University, System Health Science Center College of Medicine, USA.

3. Joseph Barber, "Freedom from smoking: integrating hypnotic methods and rapid smoking to facilitate smoking cessation," University of Washington School of Medicine, *International Journal of Clinical and Experimental Hypnosis* 49(3)(2001): 257–266, 2001.

4. Amy Renshaw, "The Real Story Behind the Nicotine Patch and Smoking Cessation," Health Psychology Home Page: www.healthpsych.psy.vanderbilt.edu.

5. Leondires, "Are Your Vices Preventing," 12.

6. Noah Hittner, "What You DON'T Know—IS Hurting You," www.dynamicsports.net 2004. Section 9.

7. Ibid.

8. Ibid.

9. Jorge Chavarro, Walter Willett, and Patrick Skerrett. "Fertility and Diet." *Newsweek Magazine* (December 10, 2007): 55–62.

10. Ibid.

11. Ibid.

12. Dana Sullivan, "Nine Ways to Boost Your Fertility," *Conceive Magazine, Volume 3, Issue 3* (Fall 2006): 44.

13. Chavarro, "Fertility and Diet."

14. Sullivan, "Nine Ways."

15. Ibid.

16. Ibid.

17. Jim Schwartz, "The Mind-body Approach to Fertility: An Interview with Dr. Elizabeth Muir," *Resolve Newsletter* (Winter, 2004): 10.

CHAPTER THIRTEEN

COMPLEMENTARY MODALITIES AND THE FERTILITY JOURNEY

As a woman starts to put together an action plan, she usually wants to know more about each of the alternative modalities and how to find the best practitioners. This chapter is designed to supplement the information on complementary practices from chapter twelve and to provide resources for how the reader can find the practitioners or healers with the right expertise to be a partner on their fertility journey.

WHY EXPLORE THE ALTERNATIVES?

As I mentioned in the action plan of the previous chapter, whether or not a woman chooses to use Western medicine on her fertility journey, I highly recommend that she *begin* the process by working to balance the mental, physical, and emotional components of her health by taking advantage of alternative modalities.

Many women—especially those with age concerns—approach infertility with Western medicine first, then they turn to alternative modalities when that is unsuccessful. Although it is a common strategy to begin with Western medicine because the "biological clock is ticking," my belief is that achieving a state of physical and emotional balance is paramount to the success of creating a healthy pregnancy. I have often observed that when a woman is out of balance, especially emotionally, many of the Western medical procedures are unsuccessful. I've worked with many women who have spent a great deal of time and money on failed procedures—because of physical and emotional imbalances—and they did not achieve success until *after* they worked with complementary modalities.

An analogy that could be used to illustrate this point is the case of a triathlete—participating in events that include swimming, biking, and running—who is not prepared. Imagine if that triathlete is out of shape, eating an unhealthy diet, nursing a bad ankle, uncomfortable in water because of an old memory, and full of stress because they are worried that if they are unable to finish, they will be considered a failure. That individual is not prepared physically or emotionally to compete. Participating in that triathalon in that state of unreadiness is unlikely to produce a positive result. If that person changes their diet, gets in good physical shape, processes their fears, and learns some techniques for stress reduction, then they will be ready.

Likewise, if a woman feels stress and anxiety, has lingering fears around having another miscarriage or being unable to have children, and has physical deficiencies from an Eastern medicine perspective (affecting the quality of her follicles and her ability to sustain a pregnancy), is she in a balanced state and ready to have a baby? Is it likely that a procedure such as an IUI or IVF is going to overcome all of those deficiencies and be successful? It is possible, but based on what I've observed over the years, it is very doubtful.

I believe that one of the keys to creating fertility is physical and emotional balance. In many cases, I have found that reaching a balanced state will often allow a woman to get pregnant naturally. Emotional balance, which I have addressed throughout this book, means processing and healing emotional issues, mitigating stress, and incorporating meditation and possibly mind-body techniques to promote fertility. For physical balance, I highly recommend acupuncture.

FINDING A HEALER

Finding the right healer or practitioner can be difficult. How do you begin that process? What questions should you ask? What resources are available?

Finding the right practitioner can be much like finding a good teacher. Some teachers can be filled with passion about the subject they teach. Some can have extensive backgrounds in their field of expertise. Some can provide an experience that is inspirational or life-changing. Some, unfortunately, just go through the motions.

The same is true with practitioners. All practitioners are not the same. They vary widely in terms of background and experience and, most importantly, the innate or intuitive ability to help clients on their journey. Ultimately, healing is the responsibility of the client—not the practitioner— but the right person can make a world of difference in guiding a woman on her fertility journey.

In finding a practitioner, it is always best to begin by asking for referrals. Many healing situations involve working with deep feelings and emotions. It helps to be referred by someone who felt positive about their practitioner and their experience. If you find yourself without a referral, most practitioners will offer a free thirty-minute consultation. It is best to go in and meet one or two practitioners if there is some uncertainty. See if you feel more comfortable with one than the other. Ask them how they would approach some of the specific issues that relate to a situation like yours. One may have strategies that indicate they are experienced in an area that is of importance to you while another may not. It may be that you feel more of a connection with one than another.

Follow your intuition and understand that decades of accumulated stuff *does* require some time and attention. The process of healing and achieving balance can take time. Looking for a quick fix in one or two sessions is unrealistic.

For some modalities I've listed in this book, finding and working with the right healer may mean traveling to another geographic location, especially for those who live in small towns or remote areas.

HEALING THE EMOTIONAL ISSUES
WITH HYPNOSIS

There have been many instances in this book where I have made reference to hypnosis because that is the modality that is designed to bypass the critical mind and work directly with the subconscious mind. The emotional issues that need to be processed, the roots of our stress, beliefs about ourselves, negative feelings and emotions, unfavorable behavioral patterns, fears, and anxieties are *all* rooted in the subconscious mind. That is where the emotional work needs to take place.

The advantage of hypnosis is that, in addition to dealing with the deeper subconscious concerns or fertility blocks, an experienced hypnotist can teach the client meditation, put together a mind-body healing program based on Eastern and Western medicine, work with cellular reprogramming, and possibly facilitate the energy work discussed in chapter ten. Some hypnotherapists may not be experienced in all of those modalities, and, in those cases, it may involve seeing a couple of different practitioners. I believe the most important part of the fertility journey is mitigating the stress response—which comes directly from our subconscious issues—so the processing of the old material through hypnosis is the number one priority in generating success.

THE HYPNOSIS STAGE SHOW

Many of the details about hypnotherapy are discussed in chapter three; however, sometimes people have seen a hypnotist performing a stage show and this brings up questions about how this modality could be applied to infertility work. In stage hypnosis, an audience is led to assume that the participants on stage must be under the control of the hypnotist because people on stage are acting silly and doing such things as clucking like chickens and singing songs. It is important to look at this situation in context. When a stage hypnotist begins his show, the first thing he asks is, "Who wants to come up on stage and be a volunteer?" Do the shy, reserved people raise their hands? Never. Do the extroverts who crave attention, have had a couple of drinks, and would be willing to cluck like a chicken even if hypnosis *wasn't* involved volunteer? Always. That is the key point: the people who volunteer are the ones who crave attention and would perform crazy antics even if hypnosis was not involved. The stage hypnotist could ask, "Who wants to come up on stage and cluck like a chicken without any hypnosis," and those same people who enjoy the limelight would probably raise their hands.

Is it mind control? If the hypnotist instructed those volunteers to go rob a bank and bring the money back to him, all of those same extroverts would immediately come out of hypnosis and the show would be over. The point is, the client is *always* in control during hypnosis and no one will do anything against their own moral code. So, the extrovert might get up on stage and belt out a show tune, but they aren't going to be making a bank run on behalf of the hypnotist.

THE HYPNOSIS SESSION

People often ask what a hypnosis session is really like. The session starts with a discussion between the client and the hypnotist about the client's goals and objectives. Sometimes this will include developing a plan that prioritizes the issues and outlines how those concerns will be addressed. When it is time to begin working with hypnosis, the first step is what is called an *induction,* which is a way of helping the client quiet their mind and enter hypnosis. Oftentimes, the induction can involve going into a state of relaxation or reaching a state where the interference and critical thinking from the conscious mind is greatly reduced. By going through the induction and entering a hypnotic trance, the client is able to bypass the critical factor and get to information held within the subconscious mind.

After the induction, the hypnotist might have the client imagine an image or situation. For this example, let's say that a fertility client is asked to imagine going back to a scene that occurred a couple of months prior to the hypnosis session, such as when she was at the doctor's office getting the results of her pregnancy evaluation. Perhaps, at that appointment, the doctor told the client that, because of her age and her high FSH of 15, it was doubtful that she would be able to conceive naturally.

The original response that occurred on that day in the doctor's office would likely have been an emotional one with many tears of sadness. If the client was asked—at that time—what was making her cry, and she was *not* in hypnosis, the response from her critical mind might include statements like: "We've been trying so hard to get pregnant, I don't know if I can do it anymore," or "I've wanted to have kids all my life, and now I won't be able to have them because we can't afford in vitro," or "I'm letting everyone down."

The response in the hypnosis session would also be emotional, but the answers to that question of why she was so sad would probably be very different. After connecting with the origins of her emotions, the answers might be: "I can't get pregnant because I had an abortion when I was eighteen, and I don't deserve to have kids," or "I can see my dad's face right now—this is just one more example of how I'm not good enough for him," or "I don't believe my husband really wants kids. What if I get pregnant, and he leaves? People are always leaving me. I can't trust anyone."

The answers that come up in hypnosis are completely different because they are *not* coming from the logical mind, but these *are* the roots of the fertility blocks for that woman. Could these answers eventually come up without hypnosis? With a great deal of introspective work, they might, but what if they don't? What if one is missed and that block is still in place, triggering a stress response in that woman's body? What if that woman *thinks* she has processed an issue, such as the abortion concern, but she has not truly come to peace with it at a deep subconscious level (which is a *very* common occurrence)? What if it takes years to uncover the information that is creating these barriers to her fertility? The point is that, in hypnosis, the subconscious mind can go directly to the blocks that need to be addressed.

The next part of the hypnosis session involves healing. For processing an issue, *the healing has to take place at the very beginning or initial programming of the issue*. In other words, the first time we are faced with an issue, we experience a response such as fear. Each time that issue resurfaces, it reinforces the fear. If we mistakenly process the fifth or sixth time we experience an event that triggers that fear, rather than the first time, then the initial connection between the issue and the fear is still in place. We would essentially be working with an outcome or symptomatic reaction rather than dealing with the true cause or origin of the fear.

Let's apply this concept to the issue above where the woman mentions that everyone leaves her: her issue is one of abandonment. If we ask her critical mind when this pattern started, she might come up with a response like: "I don't know. I think it was in high school when my boyfriend left me for another girl."

In hypnosis, the same question can be easily addressed, and the subconscious mind would probably provide several scenes in which abandonment took place prior to high school. In hypnotic age regression, where the client goes back to earlier scenes in their life, it is easy to find the origin. The real beginning might be when that woman was a little girl, being dropped off for the first day of kindergarten, a traumatic day that she had *consciously* forgotten. On that first day of school, the client took on a new belief: in this case, it was one of fear of being alone or unsupported or abandoned. It may have been a brief period of fear, because her mother does return and pick her up after school, but it is a significant response, and it is at that exact time and place that the feeling of fear of abandonment became part of her subconscious programming. The subsequent incidents of abandonment simply compounded or reinforced the fearful impression.

To undo or remove that programming, the client *must* go to the origin of where she took on that new belief, which in this case was that first day of school. If, instead of focusing on that event, the processing is centered around the incident in high school where her boyfriend left her, the initiating fear response is still in place. Addressing the high school issue might bring a small amount of relief, but the fear of abandonment program is still part of her subconscious material. The root source or initial sensitizing event is commonly missed in *conscious mind* processing, and that is why people often say, "I thought I had already dealt with that," when an issue resurfaces. The work they had done didn't go back far enough: they weren't working on the source issue that created the programming; instead, they were mistakenly working on an issue related to the source that came after or was a subsequent event that was reinforcing the source issue. *If the issue isn't addressed at the source, the initial programming doesn't go away.* That is the key. Using the conscious mind to try to identify the source programming of an issue can take years, or sometimes be a futile endeavor. In hypnosis, it can often be identified in a matter of minutes.

If this woman has a deep-seated fear that her husband might leave (an issue her conscious mind was not able to identify), that fear can trigger the stress response in her body, which, as documented throughout this book, can cause physical reactions that interfere with conception. Processing only the high school event will leave the emotional source of abandonment in place where it can be activated at any time and on a regular basis. Processing the kindergarten event removes the fear of abandonment issue altogether so that fear is no longer a part of her emotional programming, and no longer generating the stress response in her body.

So, in hypnosis, after the *true* subconscious material is revealed, the source of the programming is identified and processed. The way the experience is processed or reframed can vary widely from client to client. Sometimes it is necessary to comfort that little girl on her first day of school; sometimes the entire scene needs to be recreated with a different outcome; and sometimes the fearful energy needs to be removed from her physical body with energy work. All three of those methods have enormous healing potential when performed in hypnosis and very little impact when working strictly with the critical mind. Many times, in hypnosis, the client knows and can tell their practitioner exactly what needs to happen in order for them to release that fear response. In those cases, the information for healing comes directly from the subconscious and is especially relevant.

After the processing takes place, the hypnotist might teach the client some tools to use in daily meditation to help replace the old programming with new, more positive, beliefs. Lastly, the hypnotist will guide the client back to full awareness, where the issue can be discussed and the new information can be integrated so that the subconscious and conscious minds will be in agreement.

FINDING A HYPNOTIST

In many states, the term *hypnotist* is acceptable and *hypnotherapist* is not. This is simply a matter of legalities and not a reflection of qualifications or experience. Medical doctors, by virtue of their licensure, can practice hypnosis without being trained in that area. Since a medical doctor is usually unable to spend an hour in session with each patient—unless they were to charge a much higher rate—there is no advantage to seeing a medical doctor for hypnosis. In fact, it is better to work with someone who works full-time with hypnosis rather than someone who dabbles with it in their practice. There are two major organizations that certify hypnotists: the National Guild of Hypnotists (NGH) and the American Council of Hypnotist Examiners (ACHE). It is a good idea to work with a hypnotist who has been certified by one of these two organizations. Board certification is certainly a plus because it indicates that the hypnotist has passed the board exams, and it usually means that they have been practicing for a longer period of time.

To find a hypnotist who is skilled at working with infertility, I've included information on my web site at the Rocky Mountain Hypnotherapy Center (*www.rmhypnotherapy.com* or *www.themindbodyfertilityconnection.com*). It is a field that requires some specific background and training. Some of the major components covered in this book such as energy work, a rudimentary knowledge of Eastern medicine, a background in working with perfectionism, age regression techniques, experience in teaching meditation and mind-body healing, cellular reprogramming, and the ability to assist with the processing of deep-seated emotional issues are all areas in which the hypnotist must be competent. A good strategy when looking for a hypnotist for infertility is to ask them about their experience and knowledge in each of these areas.

Again, ask for referrals. I find that women who have used hypnosis for fertility are very forthright with suggesting this to other women who might be looking for alternative approaches.

RESTORING PHYSICAL BALANCE THROUGH ACUPUNCTURE

Practitioners of Oriental medicine work with meridians or channels of energy that run through our bodies (see figure 13.1). These meridians are associated with major organs such as the heart, the liver, the lungs, and the kidneys. When the energy flow through these meridians is open, evenly distributed, and uninterrupted, then our bodies are in balance and

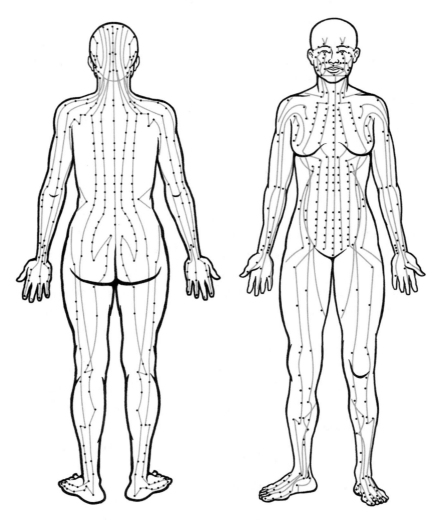

Figure 13.1: The energy (acupuncture) meridians that run through the body.

all is well with our physical health. When the flow is interrupted—by things such as stress—then the body has an adverse reaction.

For example, a patient with reduced energy or a block in the meridians that go to the lungs might have a respiratory problem such as asthma. In a case like this, an acupuncturist uses needles and herbs to restore that energy to the lungs, strengthening the lungs and the immune system so the client can breathe more easily. A Western medical doctor might give that patient a drug or inhalant, whereas the acupuncturist will try to stimulate the lung energy to function more efficiently. In this case, acupuncture is working with the cause or root and trying to create balance, whereas the drug might be focused more on controlling the symptoms.

In regard to infertility, the relationship of the energy systems to the reproductive organs is much more sophisticated. As I mentioned in the previous chapter, an issue such as poor egg quality is connected to the energy of the kidneys and is treated through the kidney meridians. When most people hear this, they ask what the kidneys have to do with reproduction; after all, kidneys aren't considered one of the reproductive organs. In Eastern medicine, the kidneys are known to be the organs that supply energy to the ovaries and the entire reproductive system. That energy helps the ovaries function at full capacity and the ovaries are then able to produce quality follicles. If the kidney energy is weak and unable to send enough energy to stimulate the ovaries and get them to work at full potential, the result can be follicles that are not viable. It doesn't mean that anything is *physically* wrong with the kidneys, it just means that they are energetically undernourished. Master teacher of Oriental medicine and author of *Obstetrics and Gynecology in Chinese Medicine* Giovanni Maciocia says that "The treatment of infertility according to the four phases [in Chinese medicine the menstrual cycle is divided into four phases] is always based principally on treating the kidneys."[1] Maciocia goes on to say that, "Constitutional weakness of the kidney-essence is an important cause of infertility …"[2] Medical doctor and doctor of Oriental medicine Lifang Liang, in her book *Acupuncture and IVF*, also stresses the importance of balanced kidney energy:

In order for fertilization to occur, the yin, yang, qi [chi or energy], and blood of the kidneys need to be perfectly balanced. When one or more of these elements is out of balance, a disharmony results and infertility may occur.[3]

This imbalance of the kidneys is commonly treated by practitioners of Chinese medicine specializing in infertility. Instead of using drugs to artificially influence follicle production, the acupuncturist is working to correct the imbalance in the body by addressing the root of the problem so the body will develop viable follicles on its own.

Since the energy level of the kidneys typically declines naturally as we get older and wear ourselves down with work and stress, it is no surprise that many women in their thirties and forties are told by their fertility specialist that their egg quality is questionable. Women in this situation can often correct this issue naturally with six months of acupuncture, thereby greatly increasing their chances of becoming pregnant naturally or with the use of a reproductive procedure. Even with a procedure such as IVF, if the egg quality is subpar, the outcome is much less likely to be successful. Dr. Lifang Liang addresses this in her book:

> A large number of patients who have tried IVF several times and were unsuccessful have soon become pregnant after Chinese medicine treatments. In clinical observation, the ultrasound shows that, after acupuncture, the color of a woman's ovaries changes from cloudy to bright and clear. The follicles usually double in number, the lining of the uterus becomes thicker, and the number of embryos increases significantly. Patients experience less side effects and feel more at ease and happy.[4]

It makes sense to correct the imbalance first—in this case making the follicles more viable—*before* investing time and money in medical procedures.

The fertility treatments of an acupuncturist are much more complex than simply working with the kidney energy. I have discussed that specific imbalance in this book because it is an Eastern medicine dynamic that is easy to understand. Infertility can also be connected to other organ systems including the spleen, liver, and heart. Energy in those systems can be described as being deficient (as in the kidney example), or it can be excessive (too much energy) or stagnant (energy that is stuck or not moving). Another factor addressed by acupuncturists, mentioned in the excerpt above by Dr. Lifang Liang, is the influence of the four vital substances: yin, yang, chi, and blood. Working with acupuncture to promote conception is a complex process, and it is important to choose a practitioner who specializes in the field of infertility and understands the philosophy and practice of Eastern medicine.

FINDING AN ACUPUNCTURIST

To find an acupuncturist, it is best to choose someone who is certified with the National Certification Commission for Acupuncture and Oriental Medicine (NCCAOM). On the NCCAOM web site (www.nccaom .org) there are tools for finding certified acupuncturists in your area. Most acupuncturists certified with NCCAOM have completed 3,500–4,000 hours of training and have also passed the board exams in order to become certified. Once you have a list of practitioners in your area, it is a good idea to look for someone who specializes in infertility.

Medical doctors can, simply by virtue of their Western medical licensure, legally practice acupuncture. Considering most acupuncture treatments last an hour, it could be very expensive to see a medical doctor for this work. Medical doctors certified by NCCAOM are rare, but do exist. You may find that the 3,500-plus hours of training to be a licensed acupuncturist—especially if that acupuncturist specializes in infertility—may be more beneficial than working with a medical doctor who may not have the same degree of training. It is a always a good idea to ask your practitioner or doctor about the number of hours of training they have invested in Oriental medicine and about their background as it specifically relates to working with infertility.

MAYA ABDOMINAL MASSAGE

Another modality that women may want to consider on their fertility journey is a form of bodywork called Maya abdominal massage or uterine massage. The objective for this type of work is to ensure that the uterus is in the correct position for conception to take place.

The uterus is held in place by several ligaments. Ligaments can stretch or loosen over time. This is especially common in women who are athletes or runners now or have participated in these activities in their past. Other factors such as surgery, car accidents, or heavy lifting can also affect the positioning of the uterus. All of these may cause trauma, which can loosen those ligaments and, as a result, cause the uterus to tip or tilt or fall out of position. A uterus that is out of position can not only greatly restrict the ability of the sperm to reach the follicle, but it can impact the quality of the uterine blood flow, as old blood in a tilted uterus may not fully drain during a menstrual cycle. Naturally, healthy uterine blood—rather than a mix of old and new blood—is essential for nourishing an implanted embryo. Dr. Rosita Arvigo, a naprapathic physician (naprapathy is a system of treating the body with manipulation instead of drugs) and authority on Maya healing techniques explains:

> When reproductive organs shift, they can constrict normal flow of blood and lymph, and disrupt nerve connections. Just a few extra ounces sitting on blood and lymph vessels can cause havoc throughout the different systems in the body. By shifting the uterus back into place, homeostasis, or the natural balance of the body, is restored in the pelvic area and the surrounding organs. Toxins are flushed and nutrients that help to tone tissue and balance hormones are restored to normal order. This is essential for healthy pregnancy, labor, and delivery.[5]

Maya abdominal massage, based on ancient Mayan healing techniques, is a non-invasive, external massage technique. The goal is to "reposition organs that have dropped and restricted the flow of blood, lymph, nerve, and chi energy ... [and] restore the body to its natural balance."[6] Don Elijio Panti, Arvigo's master teacher from Belize, says that "If a woman's uterus is out of balance, so is she."[7] Again, the focus is on balance. The ancient healing methods always emphasized the importance of balance.

FINDING A PRACTITIONER
OF MAYA ABDOMINAL MASSAGE

A list of Maya abdominal massage practitioners can be found on Dr. Arvigo's web site at www.arvigomassage.com.

Energy Work

Unfortunately, there aren't easy ways to find and choose practitioners who do energy work in areas such as Qi Gong healing, hands-on healing, and reiki. Again, the best strategy is to ask people for recommendations. A good place to start may be talking to people at alternative bookstores, health food stores, and holistic health fairs.

Once you have a practitioner you like, such as a massage therapist, ask them for a referral. Most alternative practitioners network with other healers.

If you have no luck with referrals, most major cities have publications that focus on alternative healing and those often have listings of practitioners. Again, make some phone calls to weed out the ones who don't feel right, then see a few practitioners for consultations to find the one that feels most comfortable.

Chiropractic Care

Many women have found chiropractic care to be helpful on their path to pregnancy. Proper body alignment is necessary to maintain a healthy energy flow to the abdominal and reproductive area. Women with lower back pain may want to consider chiropractic to restore healthy alignment and make sure that all energetic and circulatory channels are functioning properly.

Healing Support System

Besides the invaluable benefits of restoring physical and emotional balance with the use of complementary modalities, another benefit is that it provides a network of emotional support. It is rare that medical doctors, because of time constraints, are able to spend the time necessary to provide support of this nature. As this can often be one of the most challenging times in a woman's life, having a couple of hours each week with practitioners who can provide emotional support may be one of the most important aspects of this process. It can be a source of relaxation and nurturing that may not otherwise be available to them. While this kind of work may feel new and challenging, I have seen many people completely transform their lives by working with practitioners of complementary modalities.

In Their Own Words

Andrea originally pursued Western medical techniques on her fertility journey. In the end, she abandoned that course of action and worked with alternative modalities. Andrea went through the hypnosis process to address the issues she mentions in her account. When she reached a point of physical balance through acupuncture and emotional balance through hypnotherapy, Andrea became pregnant naturally at age forty-three.

Andrea's Story
Pregnant Naturally at Forty-three

When I was thirty-seven years old, in 1999, I underwent my first of three in vitro attempts. We had to go that route, as my husband had had a vasectomy about twenty years earlier. They could still extract the sperm but needed to do in vitro fertilization in order for us to conceive. I was a poor responder to all the medications needed to do this process, but my body did produce enough eggs to go through with this procedure. We did another IVF in 2000 and then the last one in 2001. None of them resulted in a pregnancy.

In 2003 my husband agreed to undergo a vasectomy reversal. It was successful. We tried to conceive starting in May 2003 without any type of assistance. We weren't having any success so I went to see a reproductive specialist. They did the blood tests and told me my ovarian reserve was very low and that I should consider a donor egg if I really wanted to have a baby. That's when we decided to explore hypnotherapy and acupuncture.

I had four sessions of hypnosis. In the very first session we tackled what I think was a huge mental block that I didn't realize I had: my belief that my husband really did not want to have a baby in this stage of his life. The hypnosis session made me realize that my husband loved me 100 percent and was very committed to having a baby. After that session I never worried about that again.

Another issue was that I had had a baby when I was twenty-one years old whom I gave up for adoption. Deep inside, I was certain my unresolved feelings about that were getting in the way of my ability to conceive. Since I had been able to have a baby on my own, I always thought I could get pregnant again, but I really did believe that there was something mental getting in the way and that, until I dealt with it, I was not going to conceive. I believe the hypnotherapy was essential for me in coming to peace with that issue.

I also had some ambivalence about the lifestyle changes required to raise a child. I liked my current lifestyle and was worried about giving that up. We worked on that and I was given suggestions to say every day, which I did whenever I had a quiet moment...in the shower, driving to and from work, in my daily meditation. Saying and thinking, "I am pregnant," was very helpful. In the last session we worked on what was happening at the cellular level, and that helped as well.

My objective when I began hypnosis was to try to conceive, but I also wanted to use hypnotherapy as a way to allow me to be peaceful at the end of the day with whatever was going to happen. That was my main objective—to not be haunted for the rest of my life about having a baby. I wanted to be at a place where I knew we had given our best effort in Western medicine, Eastern medicine, and hypnotherapy, and then be okay with the fact that we gave it our best shot. I had reached that point in July of 2005. I didn't think we were ever going to conceive, and I really was okay with that. I was thinking about where I could take my creativity if it wasn't going to take the form of a baby. I was thinking about travel and my career, and feeling good about everything, when we ended up conceiving! Six months after my hypnotherapy sessions, I conceived naturally and gave birth to a healthy baby boy—at forty-three years old! I feel that the mind-body work and weekly acupuncture treatments were the key to being successful.

WORKS CITED

1. Giovanni Maciocia, *Obstetrics and Gynecology in Chinese Medicine* (New York, New York: Churchill Livingstone, 1998), 695.

2. Ibid. 691.

3. Lifang Liang, *Acupuncture and IVF* (Boulder, Colorado: Blue Poppy Press, 2003), 10.

4. Ibid., xxiii.

5. Arvigo, Rosita, Dr. From Dr. Arvigo's web site: http://www.arvigomassage .com.

6. Ibid.

7. Ibid.

THE FERTILITY JOURNEY

The fertility journey is about much more than bringing children into the world. It can be a pathway to personal discovery as we challenge ourselves to heal the old wounds and experiences that have been holding us back in life. It can be the achievement of wellness and balance of mind, body, and spirit. It can be a bridge to enlightenment as we learn to let go, be in harmony with the natural world, and embrace our connection with the universe. Any healing we do for ourselves, regardless of the issue, becomes a gift to future generations, as children learn by observing our behavior every moment they are in our presence. The healing we do creates a ripple effect, because our power and influence is felt by everyone around us.

The fertility journey is about learning to love and honor ourselves, standing in our power, choosing to nurture ourselves with wholesome foods and positive thoughts, building loving relationships, having patience, accepting the imperfections of life, practicing forgiveness, bravely facing our fears, and letting go of all the stuff in our lives that does not support our higher vision of motherhood.

The path of mind-body healing is a transformational journey about creating new life, not only the life of that infant we dream of cradling in our arms, but also the new life and inner peace that comes from the heart that we have healed.

GLOSSARY

age regression: A technique where a client, while in hypnosis, goes back to an experience or event that occurred earlier in his or her life.

amenorrhea: The lack of a menstrual period.

anovulation: The lack of ovulation.

ART report: The Assisted Reproductive Technology (ART) report generated by the Center for Disease Control and Prevention, the government agency that tracks the success rates of all IVF procedures performed within the United States. It takes several years for the CDC to assimilate the information that goes into an ART report, so there is always a two- to three-year delay between the last day of the calendar year and the release of the corresponding ART report.

assisted reproductive techniques (ART): Techniques performed by medical doctors to facilitate the reproductive process, including such procedures as intrauterine insemination (IUI) and in vitro fertilization (IVF) procedures.

autonomic nervous system: The part of the nervous system that controls and regulates the functions in the physical body such as the heart muscles, digestive functions, hormone production, and normal body operations.

cell receptors: Cell receptors are located on the surface of the cell. They receive messages or signals from the environment or field and communicate that information to the cell, which, in turn, triggers a corresponding response within the cell.

chi: Vital life force often referred to as energy. A term commonly used in acupuncture referring to the energetic flow within the meridians.

cognitive-behavioral therapy (CBT): CBT can include any number of processes, including hypnotherapy, in which cognitive therapy (psychotherapy) and behavioral therapy are combined. The objective is that making positive changes in the emotional state (feelings, beliefs, etc.) will generate positive behavioral outcomes.

cortisol: A stress hormone that is produced by the adrenal glands when we feel anxious or overwhelmed. It is known to inhibit the release of GnRH, the gonadotropin-releasing hormone that stimulates ovulation.

DNA: The strands of proteins that contain our genetic material.

donor eggs: Eggs donated by another woman for IVF cycles when a patient has a diminished ovarian reserve.

endometriosis: Condition when tissue from the lining of the uterus appears outside the uterus, in and around the reproductive organs.

endorphins: Peptides that generate relaxed feelings in the body.

fallopian tube: The connecting tube or structure that runs between the ovary and the uterus.

field: The field is another term for the environment. It encompasses everything from our living environment—such as the air we breathe, the water we drink, and the influence of the people around us—to our own private world. Our private world includes such things as what we eat, how we experience physical activity, how we feel about ourselves, how much stress and anxiety we feel, and so on. In other words, the field or environment means everything in our existence: thoughts, beliefs, and feelings; how we nurture and care for our physical bodies; and the world we live in, whether that be a peaceful house in the country or the excitement and chaos of a big city.

fight-or-flight syndrome: When our bodies experience stress and the blood in our bodies moves to the arms and legs, away from the reproductive organs.

follicle-stimulating hormone (FSH): A hormone released by the pituitary gland responsible for encouraging the ovaries to produce viable follicles.

follicle-stimulating hormone (FSH) test: A test of a woman's FSH or follicle-stimulating hormone is a blood test used in allopathic medicine to determine how much effort is being expended by a woman's body to produce viable eggs for reproductive purposes. If a woman is not producing quality follicles, her FSH levels increase in an effort to correct the situation.

four vital substances: Yin, yang, chi, and blood.

gamete intrafallopian transfer (GIFT): By using a laparoscope, unfertilized eggs and sperm (gametes) are placed into a woman's fallopian tubes.

genetic profiling or genetic determinism: The practice of predicting what traits—positive or negative—will occur in our bodies based on the genetic information contained in our DNA.

gonadotropin-releasing hormone (GnRH): The hormone responsible for stimulating ovulation.

hypothalamus gland: A small gland that sits at the base of the brain and is considered by many to be the control center of reproductive activity.

hysterosalpingogram (HSG): A test to check the fallopian tubes for blockages.

induction: A technique used to help a client enter hypnosis.

infertility: Infertility is defined as the inability to achieve a pregnancy after twelve months of unprotected intercourse.

intra-cytoplasmic sperm injection (ICSI): ICSI is where the sperm is injected directly into the egg in the laboratory. It is a technique that is often used in IVF when there are sperm quality issues.

intrauterine insemination (IUI): An IUI consists of hormone treatments to stimulate follicle production and then a series of ultrasounds to make sure follicles (not cysts) are being produced. When the woman is ovulating, she and her husband go into the doctor's office. He donates sperm, which is washed and then injected through a flexible catheter directly into the uterus through the cervix.

in vitro procedures (IVF): The first step of an IVF is to stimulate the production of follicles. That is followed by the retrieval, which is when the doctor goes in and removes the stimulated follicles to be used for the procedure. The follicles are united with the sperm in vitro, meaning "in the laboratory." Lastly, the transfer is when the fertilized eggs are put back into the woman's uterus.

Law of Attraction: The belief system in which what you think, feel, and believe is what you attract to you or create in your life.

luteinizing hormone (LH): A hormone released by the pituitary gland to stimulate the ovary to produce eggs.

male factor infertility: Male factor infertility includes low sperm counts, poor sperm motility (ability to swim), or issues with sperm morphology (distorted shapes of the sperm).

meridians: The channels or pathways of energy that run throughout the physical body. Practitioners of Eastern medicine work with meridians and the flow of energy to promote healing.

naprapathy: Naprapathy is a system of treating the body with manipulation instead of drugs.

neurogenesis: A process in which new neurons grow and develop in the brain.

neurons: Cells which are present in our brains and nervous systems.

neuropeptides: Chemical message carriers found in the brain and made up of protein molecules.

ovulation: The process in which a mature egg is released from a follicle.

pituitary gland: The gland responsible for the release and regulation of hormones including output of LH and FSH and TSH (thyroid-stimulating hormone).

plasticity: Changes that occur in the connections between the synapses of the neurons. Plasticity gives us the ability to change behaviors and beliefs.

polycystic ovarian syndrome (PCOS): A condition believed to be caused by hormonal and insulin level imbalances. It is often characterized by infrequent menstrual periods, resulting in reproductive difficulties.

power of suggestion: Where an idea, concept or fear is introduced into one's belief system. A suggestion has the greatest influence when we are very young, during a traumatic experience, or when it is delivered by a person of authority.

prana: Life force energy.

premature ovarian failure (POF): A condition in which a woman is not ovulating and which can result in menopausal symptoms.

reproductive endocrinologist: A medical fertility specialist.

stem cells: A group of all-purpose cells that have the ability to divide, replenish, and become very specialized cells to repair or replace any part of the body.

stimulation drugs: A number of drugs including clomiphene citrate (Clomid) designed to stimulate the ovaries.

synapses: The tentacle-like arms of the neuron cells.

theta state: A brain-wave state characterized by deep relaxation.

Traditional Chinese medicine (TCM): The practice of Eastern medicine including acupuncture, herbs, and other treatment therapies.

unexplained infertility: A condition where infertility exists, even though there is no known medical cause.

zygote intrafallopian transfer (ZIFT): After a woman's eggs have been fertilized in the laboratory, they are transferred, using a laparoscope, back into her fallopian tubes.

SUGGESTED READING

Brennan, Barbara Ann. *Hands of Light.* New York: Bantam Books, 1987.

Chopra, Deepak. *Magical Mind, Magical Body: Mastering the Mind/Body Connection for Perfect Health and Total Well-Being.* Audio CD. Nightingale Conant, 1991.

———. *Perfect Health: The Complete Mind Body Guide.* New York: Harmony Books, 1991.

Dyer, Wayne. *Real Magic.* New York: Harper Collins Publishers, 1992.

Feng, Gia-Fu, and Jane English (translators). Original text by Lao Tsu. *Tao Te Ching.* New York: Vintage Books, 1972. Verse 22.

Lewis, Howard R. and Martha E. Lewis. *Psychosomatics.* New York: Pinnacle Books, 1972.

Lewis, Randine. *The Infertility Cure.* New York: Little, Brown and Company, 2004.

Lipton, Bruce. *The Biology of Belief.* Santa Rosa, CA: Mountain of Love/Elite Books, 2005.

Myss, Caroline. *Sacred Contracts.* New York: Harmony Books, 2001.

Northrup, Christiane. *Women's Bodies, Women's Wisdom.* New York: Bantam Books, 1998.

Reid, Daniel. *The Tao of Health, Sex and Longevity.* New York: Fireside Books, 1989.

Weil, Andrew. *Spontaneous Healing.* New York: Fawcett Columbine, 1995.

Wu, Angela. *Fertility Wisdom.* Emmaus, PA: Rodale Books, 2006.

INDEX

TO WRITE TO THE AUTHOR

If you wish to contact the author or would like more information about this book, please write to the author in care of Llewellyn Worldwide and we will forward your request. Both the author and publisher appreciate hearing from you and learning of your enjoyment of this book and how it has helped you. Llewellyn Worldwide cannot guarantee that every letter written to the author can be answered, but all will be forwarded. Please write to:

James Schwartz
% Llewellyn Worldwide
2143 Wooddale Drive, Dept. 978-0-7387-1376-2
Woodbury, Minnesota 55125-2989, U.S.A.

Please enclose a self-addressed stamped envelope for reply,
or $1.00 to cover costs. If outside U.S.A., enclose
international postal reply coupon.

Many of Llewellyn's authors have websites with additional information and resources. For more information, please visit our website at http://www.llewellyn.com.

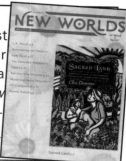

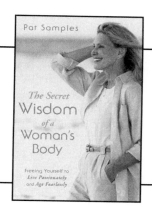

The Secret Wisdom of a Woman's Body

Freeing Yourself to Live Passionately and Age Fearlessly

PAT SAMPLES

Pat Samples counters America's fixation on youth with a revolutionary approach to midlife and aging. She teaches women how to listen to their bodies—incredible archives of our life experiences—and draw upon the emotional and spiritual wisdom within.

This life-changing odyssey begins with developing new awareness and appreciation for your changing body—the precious home for the spirit. Once you trust the body as a teacher, you can learn from childhood experiences, past traumas, heroic moments, and other personal stories recorded there. True accounts from the author illustrate how she and other women found healing and relief from grief, stress, anger, addiction, and other painful issues. Featuring practical exercises and fun activities, this remarkable guide to body wisdom will also inspire self-exploration, spark creativity, rejuvenate your spirit, and ease the fear of aging.

0-7387-1159-4, 264 pp., 6 x 9   **$15.95**

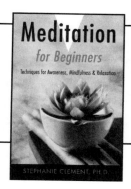

Meditation for Beginners
Techniques for Awareness, Mindfulness & Relaxation

STEPHANIE CLEMENT, PH.D.

Award Winner!

Break the barrier between your conscious and unconscious minds.

Perhaps the greatest boundary we set for ourselves is the one between the conscious and less conscious parts of our own minds. We all need a way to gain deeper understanding of what goes on inside our minds when we are awake, asleep, or just not paying attention. Meditation is one way to pay attention long enough to find out.

Meditation for Beginners explores many different ways to meditate—including kundalini yoga, walking meditation, dream meditation, tarot meditations, and healing meditation—and offers a step-by-step approach to meditation, with exercises that introduce you to the rich possibilities of this age-old spiritual practice. Improve concentration, relax your body quickly and easily, work with your natural healing ability, and enhance performance in sports and other activities. Just a few minutes each day is all that's needed.

0-7387-0203-X, 264 pp., 5³⁄₁₆ x 8, illus.   **$12.95**

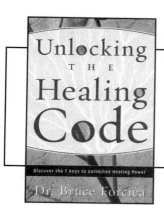

Unlocking the Healing Code
Discover the 7 Keys to Unlimited Healing Power

DR. BRUCE FORCIEA

Have you wondered why traditional medicine as well as herbs, homeopathy, and other alternative practices all work? They are all linked by a universal, mysterious field of energy that is alive with useful information. This healing information flows from the source to us across four channels, and anyone can learn how to activate these channels to heal injuries and recover from illness.

Bridging the gap between traditional and alternative healthcare, Dr. Bruce Forciea introduces seven keys to unlocking this unlimited healing power. His techniques, useful for both patients and practi-tioners, help you choose and apply complementary healing methodologies—such as creative visualization, vitamins, herbs, magnets, microcurrents, light, and chiropractics. True stories, including the author's own experience with recovering from chronic illness, highlight how numerous people have found relief using this groundbreaking program for healing.

0-7387-1077-6, 216 pp., 6 x 9   **$14.95**